Involving Families in Care Homes

Bradford Dementia Group Good Practice Guides

Under the editorship of Murna Downs, Chair in Dementia Studies at the University of Bradford, this series constitutes a set of accessible, jargon-free, evidence-based good practice guides for all those involved in the care of people with dementia and their families. The series draws together a range of evidence including the experience of people with dementia and their families, practice wisdom, and research and scholarship to promote quality of life and quality of care.

Bradford Dementia Group offer undergraduate and post graduate degrees in dementia studies and short courses in person-centred care and Dementia Care Mapping, alongside study days in contemporary topics. Information about these can be found on www.bradford.ac.uk/acad/health/dementia.

also in the series

Person-Centred Dementia Care
Making Services Better
Dawn Brooker
ISBN 978 1 84310 337 0

Ethical Issues in Dementia Care
Making Difficult Decisions
Julian C. Hughes and Clive Baldwin
ISBN 978 1 84310 357 8

Design for Nature in Dementia Care
Garuth Chalfont
ISBN 978 1 84310 571 8

The Pool Activity Level (PAL) Instrument for Occupational Profiling
A Practical Resource for Carers of People with Cognitive Impairment
3rd edition
Jackie Pool
ISBN 978 1 84310 594 7

also by John Keady

Younger People with Dementia
Planning, Practice and Development
Edited by Sylvia Cox and John Keady
Foreword by Mary Marshall
ISBN 978 1 85302 588 4

Bradford Dementia Group Good Practice Guides

Involving Families in Care Homes

A Relationship-Centred Approach to Dementia Care

Bob Woods, John Keady
and Diane Seddon

Jessica Kingsley Publishers
London and Philadelphia

First published in 2008
by Jessica Kingsley Publishers
116 Pentonville Road
London N1 9JB, UK
and
400 Market Street, Suite 400
Philadelphia, PA 19106, USA

www.jkp.com

Library of Congress Cataloging in Publication Data
Woods, Robert T.
    Involving families in care homes : a relationship-centred approach to dementia care / Bob Woods, John Keady, and Diane Seddon.
    p. ; cm.
    Includes bibliographical references.
    ISBN 978-1-84310-229-8 (pb : alk. paper) 1. Dementia--Patients--Institutional care. 2. Dementia--Patients--Family relationships. 3. Dementia--Patients--Care--Psychological aspects. 4. Medical personnel and patient. 5. Caregivers. I. Keady, John, 1961- II. Seddon, Diane. III. Title.
    [DNLM: 1. Dementia--nursing. 2. Caregivers. 3. Family Relations. 4. Professional-Patient Relations. 5. Residential Facilities. WM 220 W896i 2007]
    RC521.W66 2007
    362.196'83--dc22
                     2007026951

British Library Cataloguing in Publication Data
A CIP catalogue record for this book is available from the British Library

ISBN 978 1 84310 229 8

Printed and bound in Great Britain by
Athenaeum Press, Gateshead, Tyne and Wear

Contents

Acknowledgements

The authors wish to thank the funders of the two research projects that form the basis of this book:

> The National Lottery Charities Board
> The European Commission.

They would also like to thank their colleagues and collaborators:

> Mari Boyle
> Kate Jones
> Catherine Robinson
> Clare Wenger
> Helen Ross
> Ulla Lundh
> Ingrid Hellström
> Brian Lawlor
> Mary Drury
> Alicia Sarabia Sánchez
> Eva Rubio Fernández.

We also wish to thank Murna Downs (Bradford Dementia Group) and Helen Ibbotson (Jessica Kingsley Publishers) for their (almost) infinite patience.

Chapter 1

Family Involvement in Care Homes

An Overview

This chapter begins with three illustrative case examples to highlight some of the issues raised by family involvement. The conceptual framework for the book – relationship-centred care – is outlined, the reasons for a focus on relatives of people with dementia are explained, and the regulatory context is briefly described. Finally, an overview of the existing research literature on family involvement is provided.

INTRODUCTION

The relationships between care homes and families of people with dementia can be a source of stress and strain for all involved. Such relationships are not always problematic, of course, but we have visited numerous care homes where we have been told 'We don't have any problems with the residents – just with their relatives', and heard from many family members of the difficulties they have experienced with care home managers and staff. As the following examples illustrate, there are a variety of responses to this situation, and these can change over time.

June Kaye visited her mother in the care home twice a week, coming straight from work. She took home her mother's laundry on each visit, having been very upset at the way her mother's clothes had been either lost or ruined at the hospital she had been at before coming to the care home. She still felt that her mother's clothes were going missing, and had become quite angry with staff when she thought that another resident was wearing her mother's clothes one evening. Staff dreaded her visits, and kept out of the way when she was around. June felt that she was never informed of what was happening with her mother; she found the visits increasingly difficult, as her mother did not seem interested in the family, even when she was shown photographs of her new great-grandchild. June also felt unsupported by her two brothers, who rarely visited, although they lived close by. It was June who had been the one who had supported their mother at home since their father had died two years ago; this was when it became clear that June's mother had major memory problems, and that her husband had successfully been covering these up. After she had been found wandering in the street in the early hours of the morning, she had been admitted to hospital, dementia had been diagnosed, and the care home place arranged. June had gone along with this plan, as there seemed to be no other alternative, but, nonetheless, continued to feel guilty about her mother going into a home, and dreaded her mother saying 'When can I go home?'

Jim and Ivy Spencer had been married for 55 years when Ivy was admitted to a care home; there had been a crisis when Jim was unable to cope with her becoming doubly incontinent. Jim had been caring for her at home since the onset of her dementia five years previously. He visited twice a week, and would take her for rides in the car when the weather was good, re-visiting some of their favourite local haunts, and often having tea out. However, staff were concerned about these outings, as they felt Jim tended to be rather rough in helping Ivy in and out of the car. He became irritated with the staff when he arrived and his wife was not ready to go out; staff felt he did not appreciate how much they had to do. One afternoon when Jim arrived, he found that Ivy had had a fall earlier that day. She had a large bruise and a cut on her face. When Jim was told that no one had seen her fall, he became angry, and accused the staff of not observing her properly. He was also annoyed that he had not been informed straight away, although the manager said that they had tried to telephone, but had obtained no answer. Soon afterwards, Ivy began not to recognise him, and this upset Jim greatly; he often seemed tearful, but said little to the staff. Unfortunately, a few months later, Ivy developed a chest infection, and was transferred to hospital, where she died two weeks later. The home were not informed of the funeral arrangements, but received a message asking them to dispose of her remaining clothing.

Mrs Hussain had looked after her husband at home for three years after he developed dementia; her own health was not good and she found it very difficult when he became aggressive as he did if she tried to help him with washing and dressing. He was admitted to a large hospital 15 miles away from their home when caring for him became too much for Mrs Hussain. She only saw him once a fortnight, when transport was provided for her, as she could not manage public transport. She felt lonely and expressed guilt that she had not kept her marriage vows. When the opportunity came for him to move to a care home a stone's throw from their home, she was delighted. She was able to visit him every day, often staying for eight or nine hours. At first she was highly critical of staff and the care provided for her husband. There never seemed to be anyone around when he needed to go to the toilet, for example, and he always seemed to be the last person to receive any help with eating at mealtimes. Staff felt she was always watching what they were doing, and asked the manager of the home to ban her from visiting so often. The manager did arrange to meet with her, and this was a very useful meeting, looking at how Mrs Hussain could be involved in supporting the staff in the care of her husband. She was willing and able to help her husband at mealtimes, but had not realised she was 'allowed' to do so. She then began to help with his personal care, and gradually she built up good relationships with the staff, who appreciated her willingness to help. She would often chat with other residents and relatives, and described the home as her 'second family'.

The stresses and challenges experienced by family members in caring for a person with dementia at home have been well documented over the last quarter of a century. The aim of this book is to highlight the situation of family members *after* the person with dementia has been admitted to a care home or other long-term care facility, and to show how care homes can work with and support these relatives, to improve relationships and reduce the strain that they may continue to experience. Just as is the case for those families caring at home, the possibility of finding sources of satisfaction and pleasure in the midst of all the changes that dementia brings needs to be recognised. Care home staff have a key role in making this possible, through their support for family members and for the continuation of the relative–resident relationship. In so doing, they may also experience the reward of enhancing the quality of life of family members and the person with dementia – the aim of all good-quality dementia care.

RELATIONSHIP-CENTRED CARE

Our understanding of this situation is based on what might be described as 'relationship-centred care'. The pivotal work of Tom Kitwood (e.g. Kitwood 1997) is usually encapsulated in the phrase 'person-centred care'. Kitwood was determined to draw attention to the person with dementia, to bring them to centre stage, in a world of dementia care where their perspective seemed to be ignored and neglected. A decade previously, family caregivers had been the 'hidden victims' of dementia and Alzheimer's disease; by the mid-1990s their voice was being championed by organisations such as the Alzheimer's Society and other generic carers' organisations. Interventions and support were targeted at families, but people with dementia were rarely consulted or included in any discussions about their situation or their care.

It was Kitwood who reminded us that 'personhood' was still a possibility for the person with dementia, and that indicators of personhood and well-being could be seen in everyday situations – for example, where the person expressed their will, showed pleasure, or showed social concern. For Kitwood, personhood in dementia found expression in, and was fundamentally supported by, interactions between caregivers and the person with dementia (Woods 1999). His approach is entirely consistent with a focus on relationships.

Brooker (2004) helpfully encapsulates the person-centred care framework in four areas:

- *Valuing* the person with dementia and those who provide care for them (V)

- the *Individuality* of each person with dementia (I)

- the importance of the *Perspective* of the person with dementia (P)

- the key role played by the person's *Social environment* (S).

Person-centred care then involves the integration of these four elements, so that people with dementia and those who care for them are truly seen as 'VIPS'.

It is important to note the emphasis on the value accorded to caregivers, whether family or paid care workers, and the social environment – essentially a network of interactions and relationships, which can, it is suggested, have a major influence on the person with dementia.

For the person with dementia living in a care home, the two key sets of relationships are, first, with family members and friends, and, second, with the various members of staff who provide care. The relationship with family and friends is vital in the context of the person's journey through life; the relationship with staff is vital in relation to day-to-day comfort and satisfaction of needs. Underpinning these two sets of relationships is the relationship between family and staff, and the strength of this relationship (or tensions within it) can have an effect on the relationships of both parties with the person with dementia. This is illustrated in the 'dementia care triangle' (Figure 1.1).

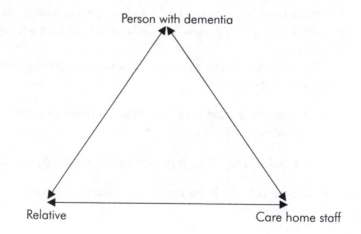

Figure 1.1 The dementia care triangle

The 'Senses Framework' has been proposed by Nolan *et al.* (2003) as a way of understanding these triangular relationships between the person with dementia, the relative, and the care home staff. Six senses are highlighted:

- a sense of security – feeling safe

- a sense of belonging – feeling part of something, having a place

- a sense of continuity – linking the past, present and future

- a sense of purpose – having a goal to aim for

- a sense of achievement – feeling you're getting somewhere

- a sense of significance – feeling that you matter.

Nolan *et al.* (2003, 2006) argue that these six senses are essential for relationships that are mutually satisfying for all concerned. For each of the six areas, the person with dementia, family member and care worker may experience these differently, yet a gap in any of these areas will adversely affect the quality of the relationship.

For example, the person with dementia may feel secure and safe when he or she has friendly, smiling faces around, and physical needs are responded to promptly and gently; the family member may feel secure when he or she feels confident that the person is in good hands and receiving good care; the care worker may feel secure when their job is not under threat, when they do not feel criticised and scrutinised for every action, and when they do not feel under threat of attack, whether physical or verbal.

This book is concerned with the many areas where family caregivers and care workers can, through effective communication and working in partnership, assist each other in achieving these senses. In the example of security, families and care workers can contribute to (or undermine) each other's sense of security. Similarly, families can help care workers feel a sense of significance and vice versa, by valuing the contribution of the other party. We will return to this framework in the final chapter of the book, as a means of increasing our understanding of relationship-centred care.

THE SIGNIFICANCE OF DEMENTIA

In this book, we focus on dementia because the involvement of families is especially important in this context. Where the resident is cognitively impaired and may lack capacity in relation to important decisions in their life, having someone who has known the person well for many years and who can be seen as an advocate for their needs is a great asset. Where cognitive impairment makes it difficult for the resident to share details of their life story, preferences, interests and experiences, having input from relatives can be invaluable in informing care plans and assisting in communication. In these and other ways, the presence of cognitive changes associated with dementia gives added importance to the contribution that could be made by family members. However, it must be appreciated that the family member may also be profoundly affected by the dementia-related changes in their relative. Seeing someone you have known and loved for many years change in so many ways, perhaps to the point where recognition and communication are lost, can be a painful experience. Many family members have cared for the person with dementia at home for long periods of time before a care-home place is sought; they may be exhausted by this process, and have lost much else besides – some will have given up their paid employment, or lost touch with friends or other family members, or given up outside interests, as the caregiving became all-encompassing.

Dementia, then, is significant because of its effects on both residents and family members. It is also the most common reason for someone being admitted to a care home, and it is generally considered that the majority of residents in care homes of all types do have some degree of dementia; this is the case whether or not the home specialises in dementia care (Macdonald *et al.* 2002).

FAMILY INVOLVEMENT IN CARE STANDARDS

In the UK, care homes are regularly inspected and held accountable for the quality of care provided, using 'National Minimum Standards for Care Homes for Older People' (Department of Health 2003; Scottish Executive 2004; Welsh Assembly Government 2004) as a regulatory framework. Examination of these standards reveals remarkably few mentions of family involvement, although each home must have a policy on such involvement: 'Relatives, friends and representatives of service users are given written information about the home's policy on maintaining relatives and friends' involvement with their service user relatives at the time of moving into the home' (Standard 10.5) (Welsh Assembly Government 2004). Other areas where relatives and friends are explicitly mentioned relate to:

- trial visits: relatives and friends are able to visit the home prior to the person's admission (Standard 4)

- end-of-life care: involvement of family and friends in planning for and dealing with increasing infirmity, terminal illness and death, and opportunity for relatives and friends to stay with a resident who is dying (Standards 19.4 and 19.10)

- autonomy and choice: assistance for residents and relatives and friends in contacting advocacy services (Standard 8.3)

- quality assurance: the views of families and other stakeholders are sought to review the extent to which the care home is meeting the residents' needs and preferences (Standard 28.4)

- complaints: the care home must ensure that relatives and friends are confident that any complaints will be listened to, taken seriously and acted upon (Standard 31) (Welsh Assembly Government 2004).

In general, the standards emphasise the resident's autonomy, and – for example in relation to contact with family and friends – stress the resident's right *not* to see anyone they do not wish to have contact with. Where the resident lacks capacity, advocacy services are to be accessed, with the potential contribution of relatives in this respect not being highlighted. This aspect will no doubt develop further in England and Wales with the provisions of the Mental Capacity Act (2005) allowing for a person to nominate someone to act for them if they were to lose capacity later, in relation to decisions regarding care, in addition to the existing provision regarding finances. Although the standards do not preclude the partnership that is the focus of this book, they provide relatively little guidance as to how care homes might productively maintain involvement of family and friends.

RESEARCH ON FAMILY INVOLVEMENT

This book results directly from our involvement in two complementary research studies conducted through the University of Wales Bangor that followed a similar theme, namely the involvement of families of people with dementia who were living in a care home. Briefly, the first study, reported in Chapter 2, looked at family experiences over a period of almost a year after admission of the person with dementia into a care home setting. This study was conducted in North Wales, and was led by Diane Seddon. In contrast, Chapter 3 provides an overview of a European project that was conducted in Ireland, the United Kingdom, Sweden and Spain and looked at family involvement along the continuum of the care home experience. Bob Woods and John Keady were involved in this project.

However, before describing these studies and their concomitant lessons for practice in more detail, the existing literature on family involvement in care homes will be briefly reviewed in order to set the book in context. Throughout the book we use the term 'care home' to refer to residential and nursing homes of all types, except where referring to a specific source or study that has used a different specific term.

Family involvement: a stressful experience?

A key finding, which provides an important backdrop for much of this book, is captured in the conclusion from Zarit and Whitlatch (1993) of a North American study where 517 family caregivers were followed over a two-year period, with 152 placing the person with dementia into a care home during this period: 'The careers of caregivers do not stop at the institution's door, but continue in an altered and still stressful way. Caregivers do not give up their role: they shift their responsibilities' (p.35). The simplistic notion that the stresses of caring for a person with dementia at home are removed following the admission into a care home needs to be re-considered. The stresses may be different, but they do not go away. Buck *et al.* (1997) report that a third of relatives visiting 'frail older people' identified in a large UK general population study, living in care homes, were experiencing significant psychological distress; the likelihood of distress was greatest amongst those visiting a spouse.

Feelings of guilt are a major contributor to the emotional distress experienced by many relatives following admission. For example, Woods and Matthison (1996) report results from a postal survey completed by 169 members of the Relatives Association in the UK, all of whom had a relative or friend in a care home. Over 40 per cent had significant symptoms of depression, and two-thirds reported feeling guilty about having to place the person in a care home. Over 80 per cent reported feeling they had let the person down at least 'sometimes'. Levels of depression and guilt feelings were strongly related. Similarly, in the large, longitudinal US study of over 500 people with dementia and their family caregivers, referred to earlier, Aneshensel *et al.* (1995) confirm that guilt feelings were intensified following the person's admission to a care home. In France, Ritchie and Ledesert (1992) surveyed 257 family members of people with dementia in two types of long-term care; 34 per cent reported guilt feelings regarding the placement, with, again, an association with symptoms of depression. Relatives of people with dementia in a more homely, less institutional form of care reported less guilt and stress. Woods and Macmillan (1994) similarly report guilt feelings to be lessened in relatives of people with dementia moving to a less institutional form of care environment. In a qualitative study, Garity (2006) identified guilt over placement as a contributing factor in decreased coping by family members after placement.

What are the factors that contribute to the effect on family members?

The home and the staff

A Swedish study suggested that 'nursing home hassles' contributed most to 'burn-out' in relatives visiting a person with dementia in a nursing home at least weekly (Almberg *et al.* 2000). These hassles included problems in interactions between the relative and staff and between staff and the person with dementia. It was concluded that, for the population sample of 30 relatives included in the study, 'degree of strain could be predicted from events occurring in their interaction with the nursing home' (p.936).

Almberg *et al.* indicated that relatives felt left out of decision-making about the resident, and were critical of the way in which staff provided care – not only what was done, but how it was done. Relatives felt they should not have to tell staff how to take care or remind them to do things. The importance of a good relationship between staff and relatives emerges very clearly from this study.

The person with dementia

It is important to recognise that in the Almberg *et al.* (2000) study family members' strain was also related to changes in the person with dementia, including aspects such as the person not recognising familiar people or asking repeated questions. In this particular sample, the findings indicated that interactions with the nursing home staff had a bigger effect.

In a study of 133 family members in the USA, Whitlatch *et al.* (2001) were able to illustrate the complexity of the linkages between the changes in the person with dementia, factors in the care home and the effect on the family member. They showed that depression in family members was indeed more likely where the family member had greater difficulty with the emotional and mental state of the person with dementia, and had negative interactions with them. However, feelings of depression were also associated with the family member not adjusting well to the placement, which was, in turn, predicted by difficulties in the communication between the care home staff and the family member, as well as by the family member perceiving the adjustment of the person with dementia to the placement as less positive.

Where the family member reported a close relationship in the past with the person with dementia, they were more likely to see them as well-adjusted to the placement. Greater support from nursing assistants, and fewer negative interactions between the family member and the person with dementia, together with the family member being less upset at seeing their relative in a nursing home all contributed to better perceived adjustment of the person with dementia.

This study demonstrates the importance of interactions between the family member, the person with dementia and care staff, and focuses attention on how the family member sees the person with dementia and his or her difficulties, in the context of their long-standing relationship.

The impact of visiting and involvement

A large, longitudinal study in the USA followed 210 relatives of people with dementia admitted to care homes for up to five years (Yamamoto-Mitani, Aneshensel and Levy-Storms 2002). Their results indicated that the pattern of visiting was established soon after admission, with 80 per cent showing a stable pattern over the follow-up period. Spouses with a close relationship to their partner before the onset of the dementia and who lived close to the home were the most frequent visitors. One group of relatives showed an increased frequency of visiting compared with the initial pattern; these were those who had been most exhausted by caregiving at home, who appeared to take time to recover. Relatives who ex-pressed dissatisfaction with the quality of care in the home tended to reduce the duration of their visits rather than the frequency.

A number of barriers to visiting have been identified by Port (2004) in a sample of 93 relatives visiting people with cognitive impairment. The barriers included practical difficulties in getting to the home (through problems with transportation rather than distance *per se*), having a poor relationship with the care home staff and having a smaller social network (of others with whom to share the visiting). Family members who reported higher levels of anxiety visited more frequently; whether this is a cause or an effect is not clear: it may well be that those who tend to be more anxious feel the need to visit more, rather than the visits themselves causing the anxiety. In qualitative interviews, family members reported that their relative's condition did make visiting difficult (although measures of behavioural disturbance were not associated with lower visiting frequency). One family member said, plaintively, that it would be easier to visit if there were somewhere to sit apart from the resident's bed!

In a large, well-controlled study of 185 relatives of people with dementia admitted to nursing homes in the USA, Gaugler *et al.* (2004) identified some positive effects of family involvement. Family members who reported visiting more frequently reported fewer feelings of being overloaded and having too much to do. Those who helped their relatives with activities such as going out and taking part in activities reported retaining a closer, more intimate relationship with the person with dementia. However, Tornatore and Grant (2002) found, in a sample of 276 family members, that more involvement with hands-on care was related to higher reported burden; higher burden was also related to having lower expectations of the nursing home and the person with dementia being in a unit that wasn't geared to the specific needs of people with dementia. In interpreting the burden associated with hands-on care, it should be noted that the proportion of spouses was unusually low in this sample (less than 10%), and that it is often spouses who wish to be involved more in hands-on care. The degree of choice for the family member may also be relevant here.

How do families wish to be involved?

Two types of care homes (nursing homes and assisted-living facilities) in the USA were compared by Port *et al.* (2005), involving 353 family members. A quarter of relatives had carried out laundry at some point for the person with dementia and a third had assisted with hands-on care. Two-thirds had assisted with other tasks and activities, such as taking the person out. Eighty per cent reported monitoring the person's finances, and 90 per cent monitoring the person's medical care and general well-being. Only a very small proportion (4.3%) of family members wanted less involvement, whilst just over a quarter would have liked to be more involved. The remaining two-thirds were satisfied with their current level, and did not seek any change. The areas where family members especially wanted more involvement included taking the person out more and spending more time with the person. Only a small proportion (around 5%) wanted more involvement in personal care.

Family members identified a number of areas in which they would welcome support in being involved. Most often mentioned was the desire for more frequent communication from the home, such as regular meetings, phone calls, more regular information regarding changes to the resident and a regular newsletter. Around one in six relatives reported a need for more responsive staff, greater continuity of care, more or better qualified staff and greater openness with families regarding any problems.

In Woods and Matthison's (1996) postal survey of members of the Relatives' Association in the UK, a quarter of the 153 respondents expressed the wish to participate more in daily care, and nearly two-fifths felt they needed more contact with staff. Over two-thirds (69%) felt insufficient activities were provided, and a quarter felt that staff often made decisions that the family member would prefer to make themselves, and that staff did not pay enough attention to the opinions of family members. Ritchie and Ledesert (1992) report similar findings from their survey of 257 relatives in France. These studies support earlier work in the USA (e.g. Rubin and Shuttlesworth, 1983; Schwartz and Vogel, 1990), suggesting there is ambiguity regarding the roles of staff and family members in some areas, and that family members' willingness to assist may not always be recognised (or even welcomed).

CONCLUSIONS AND KEY POINTS

An excellent synthesis of the research literature on family involvement is provided by Gaugler (2005), with a focus on the US literature. From this, and the above brief review, the following conclusions can be drawn.

- Families do remain involved; they do not abandon the person with dementia; they visit, and continue to visit, although the changes brought about by dementia may make this more difficult.

- Family members may continue to experience stress and burden, although the focus changes; guilt regarding placement is a prominent feature, and interactions with the care home staff can add to the stress experienced by some family members.

- Family members provide socio-emotional care; they are concerned to preserve the identity of the person with dementia, and recognise the need for collaboration with staff in order to do this.

- Family members advocate for the person with dementia.

- Some family members are happy to provide hands-on, direct care; there may be areas of role ambiguity here regarding whose responsibility a particular task is – with both the family member and the care home believing that it is their responsibility.

- Care homes that see family members as people with needs that they can help to meet are most likely to achieve family integration and good relations with families.

- There are some indications that family involvement may be linked to important outcomes for the person with dementia; e.g. in a large US study of 400 residents with dementia, Dobbs *et al.* (2005) indicate that engagement in activity by the person with dementia is higher where family are involved both in social engagement and in the assessment of the person's preferences. From the same study, Zimmerman *et al.* (2005) report that family involvement is significantly associated with some aspects of quality of life for the person with dementia.

Chapter 2

The Experiences of Family Members following the Admission to a Care Home
A North Wales Study

This chapter describes the experiences of family members during the first year after the admission of their relative to a care home, and includes brief extracts from interviews with family members. Roles and responsibilities are described, some continuing from before the admission, some new. Four stages are identified, developing over time.

- At first, guilt and loss are prominent.

- Trust may then begin to be built.

- Family members may then become more confident in relating to and negotiating with staff.

- Spouses continue to build their lives around their relative's care, whilst sons and daughters tend to begin to develop other areas of their lives.

The health of the family member, relationships (both with the person with dementia and with staff) and coping strategies were important influences on the experience of the family member.

INTRODUCTION

The first research study from which this book draws directly is a qualitative research study, conducted in North Wales, that looked at the process of admission into a care home for a person with dementia and the effect this transition has on families (Seddon, Jones and Boyle 2001, 2002). In total, 78 family members were interviewed in the period immediately after their relative had been admitted to a care home, with 29 being re-interviewed ten months later (see Appendix 1 for further details of the sample). This chapter highlights the main findings and practice implications of the study.

FAMILY MEMBERS' POST-ADMISSION ROLES AND RESPONSIBILITIES

The admission into nursing or residential care did not signal the end of caregiving. Rather, it marked an important transition point. Most family members continued to feel a strong sense of responsibility towards the person with dementia and made a purposeful contribution to his or her care:

> The care doesn't stop. It's different, but it doesn't stop.

Their contribution was often an essential complement to the practical, personal and technical care provided by care home staff.

Family members continued to perform some of the caring responsibilities they carried out prior to the admission and they also acquired a new set of caring responsibilities.

- Their *continued* caring responsibilities were directed towards protecting the dignity and self-esteem of the person with dementia and preserving their individuality, advocating on behalf of the person with dementia and contributing to decision-making. Offering companionship and helping to maintain family and community contacts were also important. Some relatives provided a limited amount of personal care.

- Family members' *new* roles and responsibilities were directed towards creating a personalised and homely environment in the care home and communicating their unique insights about the person with dementia to care home staff.

Relatives possess a wealth of biographical information on the person with dementia, relating to his or her personal preferences, needs and vulnerabilities. Most relatives were keen to share their insights and expertise with care home staff:

> I've given them all manner of information about him, how he likes to be dressed, his hairstyle, how you have to really encourage him to converse because he's so quiet, that type of thing. Fortunately they do listen, which makes life a lot easier for all of us.

This type of information is critical to a person-centred approach to care, as it can help care home staff to understand and respond to the person with dementia as an individual. It is especially important in alerting staff to the social and emotional needs of the person with dementia, which are sometimes more difficult to detect than their physical care needs. Clearly, staff should be ready to listen to relatives, draw on their experiential knowledge-base and learn from their expertise.

Monitoring the quality of care provided in the care home was also an important aspect of the post-admission caring role. This was usually described by relatives in terms of monitoring the appearance and cleanliness of the person with dementia, assessing the degree of stimulation in the home and judging the extent to which care home staff responded with sensitivity to the individual needs of the resident. Family members were often concerned that this aspect of their post-admission caring role would be interpreted by the care home staff as interference:

> I don't want them to know what I'm doing in case they get offended and take it out on her, but I'm nevertheless vigilant about her weight, her appearance and cleanliness, and I do check her regularly for bed sores.

Relatives' strong sense of responsibility towards the person with dementia underpinned their post-admission experiences, and continued to be a major source of stress for them. Most continued to feel ultimately responsible for the comfort and happiness of the person with dementia and this was often reflected in the way they defined their post-admission roles and responsibilities:

> She may have other people doing things for her, like bathing her and helping her to eat her food, but the buck stops with me. Nothing's changed as far as that's concerned.

Where the person with dementia had difficulty in adjusting to life in the care home, relatives felt under considerable pressure to try to remedy the situation.

There were some differences in the post-admission roles and responsibilities of spouses and sons and daughters who were involved in looking after a parent, in terms of the time spent visiting the person with dementia and the performance of personal care tasks. Most spouses were retired and, health and transport permitting, they visited as frequently as possible. Spouses usually wanted to be more involved in the provision of personal care to their partner than sons and daughters who helped to look after a parent. Spouses often felt frustrated that they could not do more and they distinguished between their *desired* level of involvement in the continued care of their partner and their *actual* level of involvement. In many ways, this mirrored the conflict they may have experienced in the community setting, prior to the admission, between their *willingness* to continue caring for their partner and their *ability* to provide the necessary care. In contrast, sons and daughters usually faced additional demands on their time and energies stemming from their paid employment commitments and other family commitments.

POST-ADMISSION CARING EXPERIENCE: CHANGES OVER TIME

Family members described how the experience of looking after someone with dementia who lives in a care home changes over time. This information has been used to develop a 'temporal model' (i.e. of change over time) of the post-admission caring experience. This model comprises four inter-related stages:

- breaking-in time

- learning to trust others

- building upon experience

- living with the legacy.

This model, which is based upon relatives' personal accounts, helps to predict the occurrence of specific caring demands, identify continuities and discontinuities in the post-admission caring experience and understand the changing nature of the support needs of family members. It also helps to capture the intensive, open-ended nature of caregiving.

Breaking-in time

Initial experiences in the first few weeks following the admission were usually dominated by feelings of guilt and loss. Relatives have poignantly attested to the difficulties they faced at this time:

> I was wracked with guilt, with this dreadful, dreadful feeling that I'd let him down and that we couldn't possibly get over this.

> The only way I can describe it is that it was like a part of me was missing, was gone and wasn't coming back.

> I got home after that first day and I can remember sitting on the doorstep and just crying and crying. I couldn't stop. I didn't

want to go into an empty house, see. I was inconsolable. I just felt that my whole world had been turned upside down.

Despite their best efforts, relatives often felt that they had failed the person with dementia in some way. For example, some spouses believed very strongly that they had reneged on their marriage vows. Their sense of failure and guilt appeared to be intensified where the admission into a care home had caused conflict between the relative and the person with dementia or with other members of the family. Family members can also feel very lonely and isolated at this point in time.

Initially, the admission tended to be viewed in negative terms, but the process began of redefining roles and responsibilities and establishing relationships with care home staff. This was a formative time, with relatives emphasising the importance of being able to define their roles and responsibilities in *their own terms* and maintaining that care homes should avoid making assumptions about these matters. The allocation of a keyworker can help to facilitate this process, as can a written agreement that makes relatives' roles and responsibilities explicit. Confusion and uncertainty over roles and responsibilities at this early stage can lead to duplication or gaps in care provision:

> I feel redundant when I see the carers doing things for my husband that I had done for so many years and wonder where I fit into all of this.

At first, some relatives lacked confidence in their dealings with the care home and were reluctant to share their views or any concerns they might have had. As noted earlier, they were anxious that their continued involvement in the care of the person with dementia might be interpreted by staff as interfering or as overly protective:

> I keep an eye on things but discretely. You don't want to be too critical.

These anxieties underscore the importance of care staff *actively* seeking the views of family members at this time and acknowledging their vital contribution to the continued care of the person with dementia:

> They see me as a resource because I can tell them stories about what's happened to her in the past and how that might explain how she's behaving the way she is.

Relatives' continuing sense of responsibility for the person with dementia usually found initial expression in their efforts to personalise his or her room and offer varying degrees of companionship. It was also reflected in their tacit attempts to monitor the care provided:

> Ensuring a homely feeling and helping her to see it as her home from home.

Relatives' early attempts to come to terms with the new caregiving arrangements centred upon taking one day at a time and talking things through:

> The only way I got through was to take things one step at a time. Take each day as it came and not think too far ahead.

They drew attention to the lack of emotional support available through statutory and independent-sector agencies, and they relied heavily upon their family and friends to help them come to terms with their guilt:

> My daughter was very good. She was there for me and she listened.

Their experiences highlight a major gap in current service provision. Similarly, the withdrawal of practical help, such as home care, at this point in time could be very difficult to come to terms with, especially for relatives who are older people themselves and having some difficulties:

> They drop you, just like that… Here one day, gone the next. They didn't stick around to see if there was anything they could do for me, which says an awful lot.

Learning to trust others

Letting go of some caring responsibilities and acquiring new ones were defining features of this stage. Relatives found it difficult to see other people attending to aspects of their relative's care, particularly if they have limited confidence in staff competencies:

> It tore me apart to see other people doing things for mum, the things that I wanted to do but couldn't.

At this stage, relatives placed considerable emphasis on *learning to trust* others, based on how their own personal experiences began to unfold.

Negotiating and making explicit their roles and responsibilities within the care home helped family members to allay some of their initial anxieties. However, arriving at decisions about the nature and extent of their post-admission involvement and how to interact with care home staff also gave rise to new anxieties. These included adapting to care home standards, procedures and regulations. For example, making decisions about the performance of personal care tasks, such as helping the person with dementia to undress and helping out at mealtimes, could be problematic as some care homes discouraged relatives' involvement in personal care. Some homes were concerned about the possible encroachment on staff routines, or that relatives might hurt themselves physically because of inappropriate lifting and transferring techniques:

> The staff give you the impression that they're very much the experts and so 'butt out' kind of thing. This only serves to make me more anxious.

> Like I wanted to see if I could help feed him, because they were having problems getting him to eat and he was losing weight. I was told, very abruptly, that under no circumstances must I visit at mealtimes.

Maintaining a relationship with the person with dementia was very important to their relatives. However, the limited opportunities for privacy when visiting care homes could be problematic and could be felt acutely at this stage:

> It's very difficult, especially when they're deaf and you've to raise your voice to be heard. It all feels very superficial.

> There's no privacy whatsoever and that gets me down.

> She really resents me for putting her in there and you can see it in her eyes and she can be very abusive in front of the others.

All 29 relatives found the lack of privacy stressful or very stressful, with the stress arising increasing over time. All reported that their relationship with the resident had deteriorated since the admission, and this was another aspect that was reported as becoming more stressful over time:

> At first, things seemed to get better. I wasn't running myself ragged trying to be all things for everyone and we seemed to get on better, talk more… I can remember feeling closer than we'd been for some time but that's gone now. It's hopeless, it really is.

Family members developed coping strategies to help them through the highly emotional nature of the visiting experience. These strategies include focusing upon the positive aspects of the admission: for example, the person with dementia receiving the specialist care they needed. Some relatives also put considerable effort into ensuring that their visit was a stimulating event for the person with dementia: for example, taking in old photographs and personal effects. These efforts were sometimes very taxing for older relatives:

> We'll play cards and I'll keep her up to date about local events and family news. We'll also reminisce about the good old days.

This was a time for reflection, with relatives looking back at their caregiving career to date, taking stock and finding meaning in what had happened. Most relatives reported a sense of relief from the practical demands of the caring role. However, a further challenge confronted by some at this point related to their own deteriorating health. Previous constraints on their time and energies, during the course of a prolonged and intensive period of providing care, had limited opportunities for self-care and preventative-health behaviours.

Building upon experience

Having acquired some experience of the care home setting, relatives were better able to rise to the challenge of continuing to provide support to the person with dementia and to implement appropriate coping strategies. The accumulation of essential insights into care home life, which relatives often described in terms of 'know how', could help to bolster their confidence:

> You become more clued up about how things work, and the routines they have and what needs doing.

> I've learned what's needed, and I'm more sure of how things stand.

This confidence, in turn, encouraged relatives to share their knowledge and expertise with care home staff. These exchanges could help to shape family–staff relationships and relatives' perceptions of care home life:

> Any decisions are halved between me and them, we work as a team.

By this stage, most family members had negotiated their roles and responsibilities with care homes, albeit it with varying degrees of specificity. They were better placed to identify positive aspects of the admission, which could bring some relief:

> I feel happier now. He's eating better and looks well. He's more colour.

However, family members continued to remain vulnerable to specific stressors, particularly guilt.

Living with the legacy

Family members continued to experience care-related stressors in a way that reflected the continuity of their caregiving role to the person with dementia:

> I wake up in the middle of the night, wondering whether she's sleeping and whether she's okay. I can't switch off from it. I wouldn't want to...

Guilt remains *the* most stressful aspect of the relatives' post-admission experience:

> It gnaws inside of me and it never, never goes away.

All 29 relatives interviewed for a second time reported that their feelings of guilt were very stressful. Guilt was a major stress initially, and over this ten-month period it did not recede:

> I felt guilty at first, very guilty, leaving her there... It's got worse as time's gone by and it's like I'm stuck in this downward spiral of guilt and self-blame.

> I feel guiltier now than I did the day she went there... I've more time to think about it and I feel terribly guilty about what's happened.

This sense of guilt and continuing responsibility pervaded the post-admission experiences of family members, although at this stage they usually found it easier to see other people attending to the practical and personal care needs of the person with dementia. Whilst sometimes expressing reservations about staff preoccupation with the technical and physical aspects of caring, family members had gained a general confidence in the quality of care that helped them to overcome any remaining anxieties associated with seeing other people attend to their relative's care needs:

> It was hard, I admit, to watch them doing things for her that I was used to doing. Sometimes, I was probably over-critical and this was borne out of sheer frustration. I can see that now... Now I've got more used to it and, although it's not easy, it doesn't get to me as much.

Having reached this stage, the hopes and aspirations for the future of spouses appeared to focus on the care needs of the person with dementia and their own role in providing care:

> My hope is that he'll stay as he is at the moment and not get any worse.

> I want to be able to carry on helping him and for him to know that I'm there for him.

> For my part, I just hope that I'm able to keep visiting and do my bit.

Spouses continued to organise their lives around the care needs of the person with dementia and structured their activities around the care home routine, most visiting daily.

In contrast, sons and daughters who had been involved in caring for a parent usually began to plan for the future and move on. This was a formative time for these relatives, and they emphasised the importance of being open to new possibilities as they describe their plans for the future. These plans included:

- spending more time with spouses and children

- setting aside personal time for relaxation

- returning to paid employment or devoting more time to pursuing an existing career.

Most took active steps towards moving on and instigating changes to their lives. However, sons and daughters also described their sense of ambiguity and the conflicting role demands associated with moving on:

> You can't just draw a line under it… I needed to establish a new life for myself, sure, and I needed to get back into the routine of working. At the same time though, mam's still here and I'm always going to be responsible for her.

For spouses, their sense of conflict and ambiguity frustrated any limited attempts to move on, and, for some, a sense of purpose was found in maintaining high levels of involvement in the care of the person with dementia.

EXPLAINING DIVERSITY IN THE EXPERIENCES OF FAMILY MEMBERS FOLLOWING ADMISSION

The experience of continuing to care for someone with dementia who moves into a care home can be complex and diverse. A number of factors helped to shape relatives' early post-admission caring experiences. A key factor was the *relative's own health*. For some relatives their own health problems, which had previously been accorded low priority, came to the fore following the admission. They might seek medical advice and investigations for what were sometimes very serious symptoms. Relatives' own ill-health imposed physical and time constraints on their involvement in the care home:

> You become so focused on the one person that you block out things that are happening in front of your eyes. I knew deep down that something wasn't right but I didn't have the time or the energy to do anything about it. It was only after mum went in that I went to the doctors and she referred me straight away to see the specialist.

The *relative's relationship to the person with dementia* was also important. Spouses experienced considerable stress on the admission of their partner into a care home. This was due, in part, to their stage in the life-course and the limited number of roles available to older people. In contrast, the post-admission caring experiences of sons and daughters involved in looking after a parent were set in the context of their multiple roles and commitments. These included their paid employment commitments and their commitments to their spouse and children. Accompanying these multiple role commitments were role expectations; there was a general consensus amongst families in this study that less was expected from sons and daughters in terms of visiting and involvement in the care home.

Relationships of family members with care home staff were also important. Relationships are central to care home life, shaping the environment in which people live, work and visit. Care home staff can play an important role in helping relatives to adjust to the new caring arrangements and deal with their feelings of guilt and loss. Relationships between relatives and care home staff were variable.

Positive relationships were usually underpinned by a mutual respect for one another's roles, responsibilities and expertise, along with regular communication and consultation and a concern for the relative as an individual:

> Very amicable. We all get on well. It's like going to see friends. They always want to know how I'm getting on.

An acceptance of family involvement in the continued care of the person with dementia was also important and was often depicted by care homes in terms of engaging with families as *partners* in the care process. In contrast, problematic relationships were characterised by ambiguity over respective roles and responsibilities and by poor channels of communication:

> When my husband first went in, I was told that I was interfering too much. We still have angry words about this.

> They do things and I'm left reeling, thinking how nice it would've been if they'd asked me.

Relatives' strategies for coping also influenced their post-admission caring experiences. The term 'coping strategy' describes the behaviours, practices and perceptions that family members used in their efforts to manage the stress associated with the admission into nursing or residential care. Some of the main coping strategies used included:

- talking things through, usually with family and friends

- drawing on strong religious beliefs

- focusing on roles and responsibilities in the care home

- re-framing the admission in positive terms.

When re-framing the admission in positive terms, relatives tended to focus on the practical and logistical problems they faced whilst caring for the person with dementia in the community and their sense of relief that some of these demands had been lifted.

The *circumstances surrounding the admission* into nursing or residential care also had an important bearing upon the early experiences of family members. These circumstances were defined by relatives in terms of who had instigated the admission, the time-span over which the decision had been made, and the planned or crisis-driven nature of the admission. When the *initial* instigation had come from a health or social care professional, it was often easier for the family member to accept the admission. Having said this, most relatives wanted to be involved both in the decision-making process and in the choice of a particular home. The time-span over which the decision took place varied depending upon whether it was planned or crisis-driven. Family members reported that they had more difficulty in coming to terms with crisis, time-limited decisions.

CONCLUSIONS

This chapter has considered the experiences of family members during the first year following the admission into a care home. The findings are consistent with the literature reviewed in Chapter 1, and elaborate on some important aspects. Family members feel a strong sense of responsibility and desire for involvement. While adjustment and adaptation occurs in many areas, continued feelings of guilt remain a central feature. The relationships of family members – both with the person with dementia and with the care home and its staff – are central to understanding their experiences. Finally, all efforts to support families following the admission of a relative into a care home should recognise the complexity and diversity of the post-admission caring experience.

KEY POINTS

- Feelings of guilt remain prominent.

- The circumstances of the admission are important; crisis admissions are more difficult to cope with.

- Family members often wish to remain involved: those who wish to make a contribution to the continued care of their relative should be supported in their efforts.

- Relatives' roles and responsibilities, along with those of care home staff, should be made explicit at an early stage.

- Continuing roles included advocacy and decision-making, and protecting the dignity and individuality of the person with dementia.

- New roles included monitoring the care provided, personalising the care received and offering their knowledge and experience of the person with dementia to the staff.

- Care homes must engage with families as partners in the care process and staff should be ready to learn from family members' unique knowledge of the person with dementia.

- The provision of ongoing emotional support, tailored to relatives' individual needs, is a priority area for service development. This would help relatives to consider their approaches to coping, recognise their caring achievements and begin to look to the future.

- The health of the family member is an important influence on their experience.

- The experiences and needs of family members who are spouses of the person with dementia often differ from those who are sons or daughters, especially in relation to moving on and developing other areas of their lives.

- The quality of relationships – both with the person with dementia and with staff – is a major influence on the experience of family members.

Chapter 3

Family Involvement – Perspectives from Staff and Families

A European Study

This chapter presents the results from a four-nation European project and reports on the perspectives of family members and care home staff, and their perceptions of each other. We describe the influence of the philosophy of the home on family involvement and the meaning of involvement for families. Positive and negative perceptions of each other are apparent from both parties. Important concerns for families are described and include the quality of care and their relationship with the staff.

For staff, the relationship with family members is also important, as is having information about the resident and having families visit frequently. Staff also emphasise being valued and the support of colleagues. The shared concerns of staff and family members are highlighted; these include:

- the need to understand dementia

- the need for individual knowledge of each person with dementia

- the need for activities.

INTRODUCTION

The second research study that forms the basis for this book provides a broader view across four European countries of the relationship between care homes and families of people with dementia. This involved fieldwork in Sweden, Spain and Ireland, as well as the UK, and aimed to provide a direct comparison of the perspectives of staff working in care homes with those of relatives of people with dementia living in such homes. Whereas the study discussed in Chapter 2 focused on the transition from 'care at home' to 'care in a care home', this study provides a complementary insight into the relationship between homes and families by examining the perspectives of each party directly involved in the relationship. Details of the methodology used in the study and a commentary on similarities and differences in the context of care homes in the four countries are provided in Appendix 1.

A fundamental difficulty appears to be that care homes are viewed as a *replacement* for family care, to be used when family care is not available or when family care breaks down. The concept of homes working in partnership with families, rather than substituting for them, appeared to be the exception rather than the rule in dementia care in these four countries.

Although the methodology used in each country was geared to local circumstances, a number of common themes emerged that may be used to draw together the findings across the four participating countries. These themes are shown in Table 3.1 and relate to the perceived roles of families and staff, the perspectives and concerns of each, and the concerns they hold in common.

Table 3.1 Overview of emerging themes	
Roles of families and staff within the care home	
How do families perceive staff?	How do staff perceive families?
What is important to families?	What is important to staff?
Common concerns	

THE ROLES OF FAMILIES AND STAFF WITHIN THE CARE HOME

We describe the issue of roles, and demarcation of roles, relating both to the implicit philosophy of the home and to the meaning of being involved and visiting for the relative.

The philosophy of the home

In each country, a range of attitudes to family involvement were identified. For example, in the UK some homes actively encouraged family involvement and had an open visiting policy; some imposed certain limits (e.g. open visiting, but avoiding mealtimes); and others discouraged much involvement (for instance, informing relatives there was no need to come more than once a week). In some homes in Spain, there were clear barriers to involvement: the areas where the relative could go were restricted in the home and there might be limitations on the timing of visits and on the activities undertaken, with group leisure activities being the focus in some places. Similarly, in some Swedish homes, relatives' input was welcomed in relation to social aspects of care, but practical aspects were seen as more difficult:

> It would be difficult if the relatives were to become one's colleagues.

> The staff know the routines and are used to working in a special way.

Staff expectations appeared to be clear in some Swedish homes. Relatives were required to provide all the furniture except the bed and mattress, preferably before the resident moved in. Relatives were said to sometimes need some persuasion that residents should have their own possessions:

> Some relatives are nervous about them having their own things; they think the person will be even more anxious if he or she recognises the things but not the surroundings.

It was also seen as important for relatives to leave money for staff to buy what was needed for the resident. The relatives' role was seen by staff as providing information and help when the person needed something purchased or needed help getting to an appointment with the doctor or dentist, etc.

In Spain, it appeared that relatives were generally expected to accept that the staff were now in charge of the care of the person with dementia, but in some homes it was reported that relatives could help feed the person, be involved in hair care, manicure and so on and generally stay with the person in the home within the designated hours.

In the UK, some care assistants saw communication and interaction with families as an integral part of their job, whereas others felt their role was to provide physical care for residents, and that these were tasks which relatives should *not* carry out. Care staff perceived that if they were seen to be spending time sitting and talking either to residents or to relatives they would be asked to get on and carry out some other care task. This was attributed to shortage of staff; in these facilities communication between families and the home was via the management and largely bypassed the care assistants.

Most relatives in the UK felt they had been encouraged to regularly visit the resident and personalise their room (e.g. with photographs and furniture from home) and to discuss the care of the person with dementia with members of staff. A substantial minority of respondents felt that staff had *not* encouraged them at all to be involved in the care of their relative or friend, be involved in recreational activities within the facility or communicate with other relatives in the home. In Ireland, professional expectations were said to be that families would be involved at admission and subsequently help with laundry and the appointment of an advocate for the person with dementia.

The meaning of involvement/visiting for relatives

Uncertainty about the need to ring the front-door bell of the home or whether it was acceptable to remain with a relative during mealtimes emphasises the distancing and sense of loss experienced by some relatives. Some relatives spoke of a lack of privacy or of available space (such as warm, welcoming visitor's rooms) creating a further barrier. Generally, they were unsure as to their role within the home. Although a daughter or a spouse, they saw themselves as having the status of a visitor, rather than being 'at home'. They were unsure what they were allowed to do in the home.

Family members identified a range of positive and negative reasons for visiting and being involved. On the positive side, many wanted to be with their relative, to feel part of their life, and they wanted to help out and contribute to the life of the home more generally. More negative motives included being driven by feelings of guilt, and the desire to show they had not abandoned their relative. Some relatives visited to check up on the home, to ensure that their relative was being well cared for. Some reported helping because of a fear of the resident being neglected (e.g. at mealtimes); in some instances, relatives took the resident's laundry home to wash, because they found it distressing to see clothes ruined by the home's laundry, and to ensure their relative had their own clothes to wear.

HOW DO FAMILIES PERCEIVE STAFF?

Families, by and large, acknowledged the difficulties faced by staff. There was a general awareness of the pressures on staff time and the difficulties arising from a shortage of staff. Staff were seen as having to cope with physical and verbal abuse and to deal with difficult behaviour, and often to be paid poorly for their work. However, a mixture of positive and negative perceptions was evident.

Positive perceptions

A number of relatives expressed appreciation of the hard work and efforts of the staff. A Swedish relative commented that:

> The girls are so extremely nice.

This relative appreciated receiving continuous information about her husband and what was happening on the unit. In the UK, 'caring', 'welcoming', 'friendly', 'tolerant' and 'helpful' were terms frequently used by relatives. A large majority – three-quarters – of relatives in the UK surveyed reported that they had a good relationship with the staff, felt comfortable visiting their relative or friend and were able to discuss concerns with the staff.

Negative perceptions

However, relatives also had some strong negative feelings about some aspects of staffing and their relationship with at least some of the staff. In Ireland, relatives reported feeling anxious and 'out of control' regarding care at night and early morning; they were aware of low staffing levels at night, and could not see how the staff could possibly manage. One relative commented she had never met the same member of staff twice over a couple of months. Because staff were so overworked relatives expected to have to await a response to any request.

In Spain, staff were also said not to devote enough time to resolving relatives' concerns and doubts or to answering their requests for information about the person's condition. In Sweden, time was also seen as a problem – the staff were said never to have time:

> They ask how you feel, but don't wait for an answer.

Relatives saw themselves as dependent on the goodwill of staff, so did not show dissatisfaction or displeasure. Relatives preferred to keep silent rather than complain or express an opinion. They felt powerless; many thought their loved one was neglected, but re-mained silent; many thought the person with dementia had been treated at times in a humiliating or unethical way – for example, a relative reported that she had witnessed one member of staff being short-tempered with the person with dementia.

Relatives reported feeling disregarded, in decision-making as well as in the activities and programme of the centre. Relatives also felt distanced at times by the staff's use of specialised language. A quarter of relatives surveyed in the UK felt that staff did not wish to know about their caregiving experiences, and some reported that staff did not want information about the person's life, likes or dislikes, and so on. Some staff were seen as inexperienced and untrained, apparently not knowing how to deal with dementia. Relatives felt some staff needed 'prodding', rather than automatically providing the care required. Staff were said to respond negatively to criticism, becoming defensive and turning the blame around onto the relative.

HOW DO STAFF PERCEIVE FAMILIES?

Staff were usually aware of some of the difficulties facing families, especially the emotional crisis often associated with the admission, with attendant feelings of guilt, grief, and so on.

Staff in Sweden commented that contacts with relatives took a lot of time, as they had many questions and a need to talk. They understood that relatives had a 'bad conscience' and felt their situation was a sensitive one, being both mentally and physically trying:

> Relatives feel so powerless; they can't do anything; imagine coming to see your mother and she asks 'who are you?'.

Some relatives were seen as having difficulty in letting go of the person with dementia, and their wish to participate in the caring was seen as being part of this difficulty.

Staff in the UK identified particular situations as especially difficult; these included the resident no longer recognising the relative or thinking that they are someone else, and the person not being able to talk, or showing difficult behaviour. It was also recognised that relatives may have other commitments, to family or paid employment, and that some relatives lived far away, making regular contact more difficult.

We have seen that families had a mix of positive and negative views of staff; the same was true for staff perceptions of families.

Positive perceptions

In Spain, professionals had a general perception of relatives responding positively to participation in the institution. Similarly, in Sweden, it was said that contact usually functions well, because relatives had little to complain about. They were said to be a great resource for the person with dementia. In the UK relatives were also seen as a resource for staff as well as for the person with dementia. At times they could show welcome appreciation, and also help out in the home, e.g. with feeding, washing up, helping with activities and talking to other residents – particularly those not having visitors of their own. They were seen as an important source of information, providing background context so that staff could personalise care and understand behaviour.

Negative perceptions

Staff also gave voice to a number of negative perceptions of relatives. Some were described as an added burden, disrupting routines – for example, at mealtimes when visits were said to be distressing for other residents. Sometimes it seemed the staff had two patients instead of one to deal with, when the relative arrived. Some were said to be overly critical, always finding something about which to complain, perhaps not understanding the staff's attempts to promote as much independence and autonomy as possible for the resident. In Ireland, it was felt that one factor in staff burn-out was the lack of appreciation shown by relatives.

Staff felt some relatives did not visit enough; they could understand that it can be very distressing for people to see their relative in a nursing home at such an advanced stage of the disease. Staff recognised the value of visiting for residents and would have liked to ask some relatives to visit more often but felt they could not. They commented that it can be very upsetting for residents when relatives did not visit, and staff did not know how to explain the reasons for them not coming.

Difficulty in getting families involved was reported. Staff would send out invitations and get a poor response; or staff set up a 'friends of the home' group but, again, only the same few supported the group. Staff in Sweden commented that sometimes it is more difficult to work with adult child relatives than spouses, perhaps because of family conflicts; dementia is seen by many relatives as a condition with a stigma attached. Staff felt that if relatives did not feel well, or had their own problems, they tended to take it out on the staff. However, 'troublesome relatives' were said to usually 'soften up' over time.

WHAT IS IMPORTANT TO FAMILIES?

It was possible to identify a number of characteristics of homes that were especially important to relatives. These included the quality of care provided to the person with dementia and the relationship of staff to the relatives themselves and communication with them; relatives also talked of their own feelings in this difficult situation.

Quality of care

It was clear that the quality of care was valued more than the physical environment. For example, in the UK, when finding a facility for their relative some relatives talked about being impressed by a purpose-built, well-equipped home, only later to be disappointed by poor levels of care; a less salubrious home may actually provide better care. The quality of the physical environment expected appears to vary greatly between countries as well as between homes. In the UK, most relatives surveyed felt that the quality of care was good (80%) and most felt that the staff treated their relative as an individual (77%). Relatives valued staff wanting to know about the residents' backgrounds as individuals in their own right, and for this information not to be ignored.

In Ireland, whilst relatives reported that the person with dementia was treated with respect and dignity, with more detailed questioning the overwhelming feeling that emerged was of relatives' low expectations of what should be available within long-term care. There were many aspects of the daily routine and issues relating to the quality of care which they had never previously considered. Irrespective of the type of facility, families clearly reflected the view that physical needs were met but often at the expense of psycho-social needs.

Relationship and communication with staff

Most relatives from the UK found staff to be helpful, reassuring and informative at the time of admission. They were made to feel they could continue to be involved in caregiving. Families reported wanting to know what is happening with their relative as it makes them feel they are still part of their relative's life. In Sweden and Spain, families wanted more information to be provided about the home and its routines.

Relatives from Ireland expressed feeling initially cautious with staff, feeling put off and frightened by seeing other residents with greater disability. They felt a particular need for support and education at this time; they needed support to feel 'at home' and welcome. Later they would have liked support to become involved in activities and outings, and so on.

Most relatives surveyed in the UK report feeling very much supported by the staff during visits, and where support was received it was very much appreciated, with the majority of relatives reporting feeling 'very much' valued by staff. Some relatives reported that they received support from staff when leaving the care home. If, for example, their spouse wishes to go home with them this triggers guilt feelings; the staff diverting the resident can prevent this stressful situation arising. Generally, staff in Sweden were said to mainly involve themselves with relatives through the relatives' meetings, rather than on a more individual basis. Relatives in Spain reported wanting staff to be aware of their feelings, and also wanting help regarding their loss, and to be able to face the person's death in the home when it comes. A significant number of relatives in the UK who had experienced a bereavement of a relative in a home were, however, not satisfied with the way staff had dealt with them around their relative's death.

In the UK relatives reported that they could talk to staff about things that they were concerned about and that the staff would do something about it. However, they also commented on the defensive reaction sometimes received, and it appeared that the situation varied greatly from home to home, and there were clearly some difficulties in speaking out for the person with dementia. In Ireland, Spain and Sweden relatives appeared to feel even less secure about voicing a complaint; in Ireland it was said that complaints were often only made following the death of a relative.

Relatives in the UK recognised the importance of visiting and involvement for many families and appreciated homes making an effort to celebrate anniversaries and birthdays, even if the resident was not aware of them. Here, and in Sweden, being able to visit easily was vital, with distance or transport problems sometimes posing major obstacles to contact.

Relatives' emotions

In each country relatives spoke of the mixture of feelings experienced following (and before) placement: guilt, grief, relief, sadness, anxiety. Some Swedish relatives spoke of ongoing emotional needs (beginning before the placement), such as feeling ashamed about the illness and constant anxiety. In one case the latter continued even after placement because of one resident's tendency to run away:

> You never know what could happen to him when he was gone.

Ambivalence about the decision was common:

> Sending him away was terrible.

Sorrow and loss were evident:

> You can't talk away the emptiness – you can never replace a person who's been a part of your life.

Relatives in Spain felt some anger towards the staff who would be 'in charge' of the person with dementia from now on, recognising that nobody could know them as they did. Some relatives saw the placement as positive and appreciated the greater personal freedom, but, for some, financial needs were prominent: some relatives faced drastic cut-backs when the person with dementia moved into the home, and support and advice was needed here also.

WHAT IS IMPORTANT TO STAFF?

Areas important to staff included aspects of communication, especially in relation to information about the person with dementia, the contribution of families who visited and took the person with dementia out, and the needs of staff to feel valued and to feel part of a team.

Having background information about residents

In some homes, it was reported that a pre-admission visit was carried out, where background information might be collected; staff commented they would like more access to information regarding the person's background, through contact at an early stage. In some homes, staff reported that relatives are asked to help by filling in a biographical form, helping them find out what food the person with dementia likes, and about their favourite clothes, their special interests, and any background information. In this way, the relative is a resource to the staff – their knowledge about the person is important information, since the person may not be able to talk for him- or herself.

However, it was acknowledged that communication was not always effective; in one home in the UK, background information was collected at initial assessment, but not passed on to the care assistants looking after the residents. Elsewhere, families were said not always to be forthcoming in passing on information; and, of course, sharing personal details requires the building up of trust.

Families visit frequently and take residents out

Staff in the UK valued relatives who visited frequently and took the residents out, as residents seemed to enjoy outings very much. In Ireland, some families reported taking residents out, but this was in part because of their uncertainty regarding what activities were permissible within the home. If the resident developed behavioural problems, it then became difficult to continue taking the person out.

Communication with families and building up trusting relationships

In some cases, homes had a contact person for each resident, who also handled contact with the relatives, keeping in touch and knowing the resident especially well. The function of the resident's contact person was said to differ depending on the involvement of the relatives. In Sweden, it was said that twice a year relatives were invited for coffee and refreshments (e.g. at Christmas and Midsummer). It was recognised that many relatives wanted to spend time with the staff. The greatest contact was at the beginning:

> You try and support them, but it's not certain that they want that. There's not enough time for long conversations. (Staff)

> It's a shame that contact dies out with time. (Staff)

After the resident dies, relatives are invited to the home to meet with staff, and can continue to attend the relatives' gatherings arranged by the staff.

To be valued for the work they do

A staff member from Sweden expressed a feeling that may be more general:

> You know, you can be kicked, spat at and called names. Now you can see the staff are getting tired of it. Imagine, day after day of the same thing. It's hard. In the end you can snap.

Staff felt they deserved to be valued more for the difficult job they undertook. This sense of not being appreciated was a general one, and family members were just one of the groups who were seen as contributing to this feeling.

Teamwork/support of colleagues

Staff in Sweden described how important it was for staff to support and replace one another, and talk with each other when working with difficult or aggressive patients. They felt that staff needed someone to talk with when things get too much. Staff in the UK commented that high staff turnover made teamwork and support of colleagues more difficult.

COMMON CONCERNS

A number of concerns were shared by staff and relatives. These ranged from issues around the selection of a care home, and the importance of continuity of care, to the need for activities. Understanding and knowledge of dementia and of the individual person with dementia was another shared concern. There were conflicts regarding who was in the best position to know what was best for the person with dementia, with this prerogative being claimed by both staff and relatives in a number of instances.

Selecting a care facility

In the UK, relatives felt pressured to find a suitable home quickly, especially if the person is in hospital. Generally, choices were limited, especially for younger people with dementia, and not much help or support in this process seemed to be available. In Sweden, staff considered it to be a good thing if relatives visited the home before their relative moved in, to see for themselves the level of disturbed behaviour, as this had proved difficult for some relatives to accept after the admission had occurred.

Continuity of care

Staff and families were concerned about a lack of continuity of care for residents. Staff felt that people with dementia needed to recognise those who are providing the care and that it would reduce confusion if there were fewer different staff. In the UK, it was pointed out that residents may have to move to a different home or go into hospital if their condition deteriorates, also reducing the continuity of care.

Understanding of dementia

Relatives generally wanted more information about the condition. Staff in the UK thought few relatives had much knowledge of dementia and its effects, and felt that this ignorance could lead to frustration on the part of the relative. In one home in Sweden, it was said that they used to have groups for relatives, but now had brochures about the care of people with dementia at the main entrance. It was felt important that staff could explain about dementia to relatives, e.g. in relation to behaviour changes and the course of the condition. Greater knowledge was seen as giving staff a sense of security:

> It means you can be supportive to relatives and answer their questions.

Three-quarters of relatives surveyed in the UK felt that the staff were knowledgeable about dementia. Comments were made that staff needed specialised training in dementia care; there was too much 'learning on the job', and some staff did not appear to understand the different forms of dementia. The need for appropriate training, education and specialisation was widely recognised.

Knowledge of individual people with dementia

Individual care planning was the ideal in each country, but the reality often fell short, to the concern of staff and families. In Spain, the problems of low staffing levels and lack of time meant that, whilst an individualised programme was the aim, the reality was often that restraints and medication were used to deal with difficult problems such as aggression, which would be managed differently with more staff. In Ireland, only one relative was aware of the existence of an individual care plan; personal or life story information was gathered in a piecemeal fashion, and lack of space meant there was little scope for the resident to have personal possessions. In the UK, a quarter of relatives surveyed felt they had not been encouraged at all to be involved in reviewing their relative or friend's care plan and the information flow from relatives to care staff can be difficult in some homes where the care staff do not have access to the documentation.

Staff in Sweden stated that a care plan was usually written for each resident, but was seldom followed up:

> Therefore, we don't know if the care plan is of any benefit.

Typically, relatives would be present when the care plan was drawn up; it mostly had to do with medical aspects of the resident's care, but the relatives could input information about the person's interests and background. The care plan was seen as a necessity for good individualised care, but shortage of time meant that its full potential was not achieved.

Need for activities

In Ireland, relatives were critical of the lack of stimulation on offer, often with the TV being on all day as a passive substitute. In Sweden, time was seen by staff as the factor preventing more activities; in one home, therapy had been discontinued. They felt music should be used more, as the residents seemed to remember all the words of the old songs. In Spain, there is more emphasis on activity as therapy, with programmes of psycho-stimulation, occupational therapy, physiotherapy and reality orientation being offered.

Families in the UK were very concerned about the often rapid deterioration of their relatives once they entered a long-term care facility; they thought there should be more stimulation for residents. Some relatives said that there were activities for the more able residents, while there was nothing for the less able who needed a lot of help. Staff said that there was not always enough time for activities and that families often did not help.

Expectations of care – conflict of who knows best

In Sweden, as mentioned previously, there was concern over relatives' involvement in practical aspects of care. In Spain, the issue of who is now in charge of the person who has been cared for at home was raised, with the implication that the home's routines and policies now take precedence. This theme emerged in each country, with homes and relatives finding it difficult to make an equal partnership. This is perhaps shown most clearly in the staff comment highlighted previously that relatives' desire to continue to be involved in care was a reflection of their difficulty in 'letting go'.

CONCLUSIONS

A clear picture emerges from the fieldwork in four European countries, with a variety of types of residential provision and differences in level of family involvement. The relationship between relatives and care staff, which initially comes into being for the benefit of the resident with dementia, is one that has the potential to benefit all parties involved. If it works well, then the relative will have a more fulfilling, and possibly less stressful, involvement; staff will enjoy an additional resource and greater job satisfaction; and residents will benefit from co-ordinated efforts to provide person-centred care. It is evident that, unfortunately, often the relationship is characterised by tensions, misunderstandings, misperceptions and poor communication, and runs the danger of neither relative or staff member feeling valued by the other, and the resident's needs being, therefore, less well met.

The relationship is clearly a complex one. It is unlikely that there is a single formula that would improve it. Relatives will vary greatly in how much they are able or wish to be involved; it would be inappropriate to pressurise a relative into visiting, when perhaps they feel they have done their grieving already for what they have lost. Each resident–relative relationship is unique, and what has gone before will shape the relative's current feelings for the person. However, if lines of communication could be opened up between relatives and staff, and each helped to see and appreciate the other's perspective, then, perhaps, staff and relatives could begin to work on improving their relationship, and find ways of supporting and valuing each other. The aim of the next three chapters of this book is to provide pointers as to how this process can be encouraged – not to prescribe what should happen but, rather, to illustrate the variety of ways in which constructive partnerships can be developed and maintained.

KEY POINTS

- Care homes vary greatly with regard to the extent they encourage and support family involvement.

- Family members are often uncertain about what they are permitted to do in the care home.

- There are clear tensions in the relationship between relatives and care staff; family members often feel disregarded, and that staff react defensively; care staff feel families could visit more often and be less critical; there is sometimes conflict about who knows what is best for the person with dementia.

- The quality of relationship and communication was important to both parties; each wanted to be valued by the other.

- Family members often have needs for emotional support; where support was offered by staff, this was much appreciated and contributed to a good, trusting relationship.

- Family members and staff wanted care to be personal and individualised and recognised the need for more activities.

- Family members and staff recognise that there is a need for all concerned to have a greater understanding of dementia.

Chapter 4

Family Involvement
Guidelines and Good Practice

This chapter provides practical guidance for care home staff regarding the variety of ways in which families can be involved in the life of the person with dementia in the care home. Ways of making visits less difficult, practically and emotionally, for relatives are discussed. Three key areas of family involvement are described:

- monitoring the care provided

- advocacy and decision-making for the person with dementia

- providing care, outside the home or within it.

Ways in which staff can support families who choose to become involved in these roles are also detailed.

INTRODUCTION

It is apparent from the evidence discussed in the previous chapters that there are a number of aspects of caregiving that may continue – perhaps in a slightly different fashion, or develop anew – following the admission of the person with dementia to a care home. As we have seen, there is wide variation in the extent to which the continued role of the family member is discussed (or encouraged) at this time.

If the family member has been under great stress, it is not surprising that those around them emphasise the opportunity for 'a rest'. Some may even advise the caregiver not to visit at first, so the person with dementia can 'settle in' – well-intentioned advice, but possibly misplaced as it can lead to a situation where one day the relative was providing all the love and support whereas the next day it is the care home that has taken over this role. From the relative's perspective, this may make them feel redundant and unwanted. Whilst families may well have been finding the situation difficult and stressful, for some relatives this may well reinforce feelings of helplessness, failure and guilt. To switch from round-the-clock input to occasional visits may be too dramatic a change and the nature and level of involvement needs to be carefully negotiated with families from the outset.

Many family members would want continued involvement, but are uncertain what is possible, even what is allowed. For most, this will be a new experience, and they will rely largely on the information given by the care home and by professionals involved in the admission. Caregiving relationships are typically long-standing, and for all concerned it is very important that these relationships (between people with dementia and their relatives and friends) are maintained after admission, particularly where those relationships have been very close. The most direct and effective way of maintaining these relationships is to remove barriers and obstacles to the continued involvement of families in caregiving.

In this chapter, we describe some of the ways in which families can be, and have been, involved in care homes; it is important that the potential for involvement is more widely recognised, so that relatives are not left wondering 'How do I fit in?', 'What can I do?', 'Will I have a role?' Family involvement need not be limited to the traditional view of visiting. There are a variety of levels and types of involvement that families may wish to have, and facilities have much to gain from welcoming and encouraging such participation.

There needs to be acceptance that different relatives have different preferences and needs, and that not all will want to be involved in the same way. There is, in fact, a range of ways in which families can contribute to the resident's life in the home; this is the focus of this chapter. Essentially, from the relative's perspective, these involve:

- monitoring the care provided

- acting as advocate for the person with dementia

- ensuring that the care received is personalised.

These roles reflect a significant change from the position that relatives would have occupied in past times, when they would simply have been 'visitors' – a contact with the outside world, but little more than peripheral to the smooth running of the 'institution' and not central to its purpose. Thankfully, this philosophy has now changed. Before considering the ways in which relatives can be involved, we will examine the obstacles to relatives engaging with the care home and approaches that may be helpful in overcoming these.

RELATIVES OR VISITORS?

Traditionally, visiting in, say, a hospital environment was strictly controlled. It could only occur at times to suit the ward environment, outside mealtimes and ward rounds. A notice at the entrance to the ward would announce visiting times and a bell would ring to signal the time for all friends and family to leave. The number of visitors was also limited, reinforced by an absence of chairs available for visitors to use. On the typical open ward, there was no privacy with every conversation heard by those in the surrounding beds. Children and pets were most definitely not welcome!

Times have changed, and, in any case, a care home does not operate under some of the constraints of a hospital ward. There is the opportunity in the care home to do things in a very different manner. Relatives are no longer seen simply as a barely necessary nuisance, an intrusion, but rather as a resource and as care partners – in fact, as valued members of the team.

This begins with the welcome that the relative receives; of course, it's not always possible for a long conversation at the moment the relative arrives, but a friendly greeting makes all the difference. There is an open visiting policy, visiting hours are not restricted, and those relatives who enjoy helping the person with dementia with their meal are positively encouraged to visit at mealtimes. No bell is rung to dismiss the relatives from the premises; they are encouraged to feel at home, relaxed and comfortable in the home. The more 'homely' the care home environment is, the more possible this will be as it is difficult for the layperson to feel comfortable in a clinical environment.

There is recognition that visiting is not easy for some relatives. A number of relatives have poor health and their mobility may be restricted. They may not have their own transport and the home may not be readily accessible to them by public transport. There are parts of the UK where the nearest suitable care home is an 80-mile round trip from the person's home, with poor public-transport links. A care home that encourages the involvement of relatives will take steps to help relatives in such a position; for example, the home could make available a list of relatives who are prepared to share cars or taxis with other relatives in need of transportation; or it could produce a list of low-cost voluntary transport schemes that may be available for relatives who have health problems or disabilities. Where relatives come from a long distance, some homes make it possible for them to stay in the home in some circumstances.

Visiting may be difficult in practical terms, but it can also be demanding and emotionally draining for relatives, particularly perhaps when feelings of guilt and loss are strong. Care home staff can recognise these feelings and their impact, and learn to identify some of the situations that can serve to make these feelings worse. For example, it can be very difficult for a relative if the person with dementia becomes very upset as the relative leaves – perhaps because they find it difficult to understand why they are not leaving with them. The support of a sensitive member of staff at this time can make all the difference to the parting; the staff member is able to engage the person with dementia, so that they do not feel abandoned and alone when their relative leaves. There may still be tears at times – that is, after all, a normal part of the human experience of parting from a loved one – but the relative and person with dementia are not left to cope alone, unsupported.

Many relatives feel a sense of responsibility for the person's behaviour; if they are greeted with a member of staff informing them that the person with dementia has been aggressive – perhaps lashing out at a member of staff or another resident – this may add to their sense of guilt. Discussion of such matters needs to be in a supportive context, where all the needs of the person with dementia are discussed, and the various factors that might lead to such an episode can be considered; these might, for example, in this instance include: the physical health of the person with dementia, such as an infection or a change of medication; the approach of others (a new member of staff, say, who approached the person from behind, and so was perceived as a threat, with the person lashing out in self-defence); and frustration, perhaps at a failure to complete a task that was previously very easy for the person.

The relative may feel a strong sense of loss, and will be much more aware than staff in the home of just how much the person with dementia has changed, of how different they now are, from five or ten years ago, say. Relatives sometimes express this loss with phrases such as 'My husband has gone – it's still his body, but not the man I married', or 'It's like a living death, the body remains but the mind has gone'. Staff, on the other hand, should be trained to recognise the indications of the person as a person that remain: Kitwood (1997) describes how personhood need not be lost in dementia, but that it is very much up to those around the person with dementia to uphold and maintain it. Relatives, with their in-depth knowledge of the person's life story, personality, lifestyle, interests, preferences and choices, have a key role in supporting the identity of the person with dementia.

Staff can help relatives to recognise the importance of their potential contribution by ensuring they mention the positive aspects of the person's skills and behaviour. As mentioned, it can be devastating, for example, when the relative feels that the person with dementia no longer recognises them; if a member of staff is able to point out that only yesterday the person with dementia was talking about the relative, or that their eyes lit up when they were told the relative would be coming today, this can help the relative feel the relationship is still a two-way process. Staff who become skilled in noticing these small indications of interest, recognition and well-being, and take the trouble to pass them on to the relative, can help support the personhood of the person with dementia.

Visiting is also easier when the flow of information is good. For example, the fact that as the relative comes into the home there is an accurate, up-to-date noticeboard, containing today's menu, a programme of planned activities and the names of members of staff currently on duty can be a great help in orientating the relative and reducing uncertainty.

Many homes offer somewhere private for relatives to meet with the person with dementia. Where the person has his or her own room, this may be suitable; or there may be a comfortable room set aside for the purpose. With an open-visiting policy, no restrictions are placed on the numbers of relatives and friends visiting; if there are concerns regarding the person with dementia being overwhelmed, then the home needs to arrange a meeting with the key relatives to discuss how visits could be spaced better. In some homes, it is common for families to have the use of a large room for a family celebration to mark a special birthday or anniversary for the person with dementia or their spouse.

Open visiting also means that children are welcome; of course, parental supervision is required, but there are few better ways of bringing to life the dayroom of a care home than the presence of a small child. Grandparenting skills surface once again, and all eyes in the room follow the antics of the child; nothing is more natural than the child and person with dementia joining in a game together, although it may not be clear who is helping who. Pets can also be welcomed, although supervision and planning may be required depending on the size and energy of the animal involved!

Some homes are able to accommodate residents' pets when they enter the home (usually 'within reason'), but, even where this is not possible, a visiting pet, under control, provides a certain source of stimulation to all the residents present.

The key features of the care home that involves family members are that it affirms the value of visiting and provides support for relatives in relation to the practical and emotional obstacles that may arise. Staff in the home take steps to ensure that relatives feel valued and included and that they are well informed regarding what is happening generally in the home, and specifically in relation to the person with dementia.

RELATIVES AS MONITORS OF CARE

> I think it's really really important that relatives or visitors are keeping an eye on what's going on… I do feel now that my role is to keep going in there to make sure that he and others really are looked after. (Relative)

People with dementia need their care to be provided in a respectful and dignified way, with their preferences and usual routines being respected and their abilities promoted. Through regular visits, relatives are in a good position to observe whether or not the staff are caring for the 'whole person', not just the resident's physical needs. For example, families will want to see their relative with dementia wearing his or her own clothes. The home should encourage families (including the person with dementia, where possible) to comment from the beginning about their satisfaction with the person's care, and then address any causes of concern or complaint. In any care home, there is room for improvement and for enhancing the quality of care; a good home will be open about this and will welcome comments and complaints, recognising that this type of feedback is essential in developing a higher standard of care. Managers of such homes will ask relatives how happy they are with the home, even months and years after admission, and make themselves available to discuss and address problems.

It is important that relatives know what they can expect from the staff in terms of the care they can provide. Some relatives feel that their loved ones should be receiving the sort of one-to-one care that they had when they lived at home. With scarce resources, this is often not the reality. Staff may have little time for taking residents for walks or participating in other forms of recreation. People who need help with feeding might have to wait for their meal, and food sometimes gets cold. Cleaning in the home may have been cut down. Laundry is often handled in a routine way and not always at the right temperature. Staff need to be open with relatives about standards of care within the home. Through talking to relatives about their expectations and making it possible for them to get involved, relatives can help to raise these standards themselves. Inspection arrangements for care homes are increasingly likely to canvas opinions and views from family members, and this provides an important mechanism for relatives to comment on their experience of the home, both positive and negative features.

RELATIVES AS ADVOCATES

Relatives, especially those who provided day-to-day care at home, can feel that they have lost control over what happens to the person with dementia when he or she moves into a home. Spouses, in particular, can feel that they are pushed away from their rightful role as protector and proxy for their husband or wife. As partners in care, however, relatives are not deprived of this role. Instead, staff and relatives work together to ensure that the care provided is in the best interests of the resident.

As the disease progresses, people with dementia often lose the ability to express themselves adequately. Relatives therefore have a very important advocacy role to play, representing the interests of the resident to the staff. Relatives should therefore be consulted about any changes in the resident's care (e.g. medication, plan of care, hospitalisation). The relative may wish to accompany the person on hospital visits, and so on. In this way, families still feel that they have some part to play in what happens to their relative, and that they are not excluded from decision-making once the person with dementia has moved into long-term care. Of course, the person with dementia should also be consulted appropriately when decisions need to be made. Both relatives and staff should try to determine the resident's wishes about current and future care while he or she is still able to communicate an opinion to others.

This advocacy role means that relatives would be involved in drawing up and reviewing the resident's plan of care and that their views would be respected just as much as any other member of the care planning team; they can expect to be spoken to honestly and realistically. The important people in the resident's social network would be recognised and relatives or friends involved in regular reviews. Not all the person's relatives may be in agreement about the person's care, and so there needs to be mechanisms for respecting such differences, and resolving them where possible. This will include the involvement of an independent advocate for the person with dementia where family differences make it difficult for one relative to act as advocate.

When the person's health deteriorates to the point where he or she appears to be entering a terminal phase, families need to be fully involved in discussions regarding the management of the person's condition. Questions of treatment – such as those around resuscitation or the use of antibiotics in the case of pneumonia – should have been discussed previously with the doctor so that everyone is aware of what is to be done. Death is the only certainty in life, and quality of life is underpinned by assurance that, as death approaches, the person's comfort and well-being will be maintained, and that they will be close to and supported by those whom they know and love. The resident's family may wish to be involved in simple care tasks during this terminal phase. Whenever possible, a relative should be able to remain with the person with dementia for as long as he or she wishes. It is very helpful when a home is able to offer relatives a bed to stay overnight, especially when the resident is very ill or when death is near. These end-of-life issues are discussed in more detail in Chapter 6.

RELATIVES AS CAREGIVERS

> We're encouraged to help…like they were short-staffed a few weeks ago, I went down to feed my mother three times a day to help them. *But I enjoyed it.* And we can help with other residents… There's a lot that don't have families visiting, so we sit and talk to them. (Relative)

There are a number of ways that caregiving can continue after the admission to the care home, from hands-on care (such as feeding or helping the person with grooming etc.) to companionship and sitting talking with the person.

Helping outside the home

There are some caregiving activities that can be carried out between visits to the home. Some relatives continue to look after the person's financial affairs, ensuring bills are paid and that the person's savings are well looked after. Some will go shopping for the person, perhaps now able to do this in a more relaxed fashion than when the person was at home; new clothes and other personal items for the person may be purchased. Some relatives even take the person's laundry home for them on a regular basis, preferring to look after the person's clothes in this way, rather than entrusting them to a communal laundry service.

Helping the person feel at home

Relatives can be encouraged and helped to personalise the resident's room with photographs, furniture and other favourite possessions. Even if the person with dementia does not have his or her own room, pictures can be placed on a wall or bedside locker, and the bed made up with the resident's own bedding. Personal items can be used to assist with reminiscence work. They are valuable in reminding staff of the person's life story, interests and achievements. Furnishing rooms in this way also helps to make the environment more homely. In some homes, relatives are encouraged to be involved in decorating the room to the person's

taste. A number of families have produced albums of clearly
labelled photographs, as a 'This is your life' book, setting out
clearly and simply some of the key aspects of the person's life to
date. Such a book can be a great help to staff in getting to know the
person, as well as helping maintain the identity of the person with
dementia. It is already possible for families to create a CD or DVD
containing the person's photographs, music and video-clips for the
same purpose, although more help and support in using this may be
required.

Outings

Some relatives enjoy taking their loved one out, and this can really
be appreciated by the person with dementia, who may feel cut off
from the world outside the home. A trip to a favourite place, be it a
beauty spot, a garden centre or a pub, encourages memories and
conversation; the journey itself is enjoyed by some. Staff can give
practical support to relatives who would like to take the person
with dementia out. This might include, for example, a supply of
medication or continence aids; use of a wheelchair; or even a member of staff to help take the resident out.

Sometimes relatives want to take the person home for the day,
for a family meal, perhaps. However, they might be concerned
whether the person would then refuse to go back to the home and
that an enjoyable day might therefore end with distress and unhap-
piness. Here the staff from the home can help the relative in
considering how likely this is to happen: does the person return
happily from other trips out? Are they always asking to go home?
Could a member of staff or another trusted helper be available to
help bring the person back, if needed?

Group outings are organised by some homes, perhaps taking
out a small group on a mini-bus. For example, one care home in
London organised a bus trip each year to see the Christmas lights.
Another care home hired a room in a pleasant pub for a Christmas
party for residents and families.

Activities in the home

Taking part in activities with the person with dementia in the home can also be valuable. These might include, for example, games of cards or dominoes, art and music sessions, looking through photograph albums. Pets and children can also be sources of interest and meaningful activity. Having a shared interest or activity helps communication and makes visiting less demanding for the relative, making it easier to find topics of conversation. Activities should be meaningful to the person with dementia (enabling the person to use his or her skills and abilities, and avoiding failure) and enjoyable for their relative (so that coming back is looked forward to).

Many homes have an activity organiser, and what they are able to achieve is greatly enhanced when relatives are involved, to assist the people with dementia in remaining engaged with the activity. Exercise and movement-to-music sessions are increasingly popular, with arm-chair exercises available for the less mobile; again, the involvement of relatives in the session encourages residents to participate, and makes the session leader's task much easier.

Relatives may also like to be involved in special events organised by the home, in addition to the group outings mentioned above, such as musical events and parties. One care home organises a monthly fish and chip supper, with entertainment provided – an excellent opportunity for families, staff and residents to meet socially. Involvement on this level helps relatives to feel an integral part of the home, strengthening relationships with residents, staff and other families. In some cases, events may be jointly organised by relatives and staff. It also helps staff by providing an 'extra pair of hands' and may, in particular, be beneficial to those residents who do not have visitors. The staff can help to encourage such involvement by ensuring that families know about any events taking place and that they are welcome to participate. Relatives can be kept informed of what is happening in the home by means of a newsletter and by the posting of a weekly timetable of events and activities on a noticeboard for relatives and residents, with advance warning of special events.

Mealtimes

These can be important family and social events, a time when everyone gets together. Some relatives like to bring favourite foods into the home for the person with dementia, and this can be helped where the home provides separate refrigerator space for these favourite foods for the resident. In some homes it is possible for relatives to be able to have a meal with the resident. In many homes, relatives are able to make drinks for the person with dementia and themselves, as they would have done at home. Some residents are able to return home for a special family meal; for others, space at the home needs to be provided for a family celebration (preferably not in a large dining room with lots of other people around).

Hands-on care

> I try to get there at mealtimes because he can't feed himself… but I feel also that it releases a member of staff from being with him for that three-quarters of an hour to see to all the others who are needing attention, because he'll need sole attention. And they're very good – I've been there unexpectedly and I have found one of them with him, feeding him. (Relative)

If the relative was providing care for the person with dementia at home before the person was admitted, he or she will have been undertaking many of the tasks that staff now carry out. Some relatives wish to remain involved in direct caregiving, continuing with particular tasks they may have found enjoyable or fulfilling. Where the person has lost the ability to feed themselves, some relatives are happy and able to feed the person on a regular basis. Many relatives enjoy helping with other aspects of personal care, such as arranging hairdressing, shaving, cutting nails and helping with make-up. These are practical ways for relatives to express love and care, helping to maintain the resident's dignity, individuality and self-esteem.

It is important that relatives do not feel excluded by staff stepping in and saying 'it's our job now to do that, leave it to us'. Sometimes staff may be reluctant to let relatives help with hands-on care tasks, feeling that they will disrupt routines (such as those around mealtimes). In homes where relatives are actively encouraged to help, staff see relatives as a resource, not a hindrance. They appreciate any help that they get as it frees up some of their time to see to another resident. In many facilities, staff find that they do not have as much time as they would like to spend with individual residents. Relatives can be an invaluable source of help in providing the one-to-one care that people with dementia need.

It is perhaps in relation to personal care that most tensions arise between staff and relatives. It can be difficult for staff to stand back, and they may be concerned as to what might happen if anything went wrong – would they be blamed? This is where the home needs a consistent philosophy regarding the involvement of relatives in personal care, which provides a clear framework to give staff and relatives confidence. Sometimes there is a clash of 'expertise', where the relative is seen as delivering personal care in the 'wrong' way. Although the staff of the home have expertise in personal care, backed up by qualifications and training, it is the relative who is truly the expert in the care of this specific person with dementia, having provided care for perhaps several years, day in, day out, before the person's admission. What is needed is open communication in such instances; if the relative were doing something potentially harmful, they would typically want to know; sometimes staff, on the other hand, have to recognise that there is more than one way of providing care, and if it works for this relative and this person with dementia it should be accepted agreed and documented.

CONCLUSIONS

This chapter has set out some of the ways in which families can be involved in care homes for people with dementia. Each relative will have a unique relationship with the person with dementia and their circumstances will vary greatly, so there is no one pattern of involvement that will or should suit everybody. Care homes need to respond flexibly, and ensure they provide an environment that welcomes and embraces family members, rather than keeping them at the periphery. Care homes also need to recognise that there are practical and emotional barriers that can get in the way of the involvement that some family members would want and that they as care homes have a role to play in overcoming some of these barriers. We close the chapter by providing a checklist (see Box 4.1) that can be used to check the degree to which a care home involves families in the care of the person with dementia.

Box 4.1 Checklist of family involvement in a care home

The following checklist may be used to review family involvement in a care home. If the answer to any of the questions is 'no', possible solutions need to be considered.

Are relatives invited to participate in activities, events and outings that are organised by the home?

Are relatives allowed to help with hands-on care tasks (e.g. feeding the person with dementia)?

Do staff feel relaxed about relatives' involvement in various aspects of care?

Does the home invite relatives to comment on their satisfaction or dissatisfaction with the care provided?

Are relatives always consulted when decisions need to be made about the care of the person with dementia?

Does the home make it easy for relatives to stay overnight if they feel they need to?

KEY POINTS

- Relatives can be a great resource and they should be considered as 'part of the team' – an 'expert' on the individual person with dementia.

- In addition to providing invaluable contributions to social aspects of care, many relatives wish to continue to help with hands-on care tasks – not to replace staff but as an expression of concern and affection.

- Contributing to tasks such as brushing hair, cutting fingernails or feeding can provide valuable functions for both the relative and the person with dementia: helping to maintain the relationship, maintaining the person's dignity and identity, and enabling the relative to feel involved in caring.

- Relatives should expect to be consulted when decisions need to be made about the care of the person with dementia.

- Relatives have an important role to play in monitoring care, and their concerns should be treated seriously by the home.

Chapter 5

Communication with Families
A Relationship-Centred Approach

In this chapter we consider the essentials of communication, and how these apply to this particular set of relationships. The need for a two-way exchange and sharing of information is emphasised, and the type of information required by each party is considered. Ways in which staff can support family members in relation to their emotional needs are described. Finally, consideration is given to those situations where family and staff do not see eye to eye, where there is disagreement, conflict and complaint.

INTRODUCTION: THE IMPORTANCE OF COMMUNICATION

All worthwhile relationships need to be worked at; good communication is essential to developing and maintaining any relationship, and problems in relationships can often be traced to misunderstandings and lack of communication. In our research in care homes we came across repeated examples of a need for greater understanding of the other party in the relationship. Staff often found it difficult to put themselves in the shoes of family members, and family members had limited appreciation of the perspective of the care home staff. Communication between care homes and families is clearly not easy; it is complicated by a number of factors.

- There is a built-in imbalance; the care home staff are on their home ground, their familiar territory, whereas the family member is a visitor, initially unused to the routines and procedures of care homes.

- There are many staff in the care home; family members have a number of people to get to know, and there may be a lack of continuity, with different staff on duty each time the relative visits.

- There are many family members who may visit a care home; with limited contact it can be difficult for staff to get to know each one well, especially where a resident has several family members who may have different views and opinions regarding the care of the person with dementia.

- Staff have to consider the needs of all the residents, which may require balancing different priorities at any particular time; the family member typically has the needs of their own relative uppermost in their minds.

- Family members may be experiencing distress related to the changes in the resident, and perhaps feelings of guilt that they are no longer able to provide care at home.

- Staff may feel under pressure, in a demanding, under-valued work role, perhaps experiencing stressors in their life outside work, in family or other relationships.

Communication is not simply about how one member of staff builds a relationship with one family member, important though that is. It is about the welcoming atmosphere of the home, the commitment to working alongside families demonstrated by senior staff and management, and having structures that make communication and sharing of information easy.

Good communication will contribute to a good-quality relationship by helping each party to understand the other party's perspective, and enabling differences to be discussed and, where possible, resolved. It will be respectful, recognising the expertise of the family member and that each party has much to learn from the other. A good relationship will improve the quality of care, by helping relatives to act in an advocacy role for the resident, and by ensuring that the important information that the relative has (which can make such a difference to the individualisation and personalisation of care) is shared with those staff involved in hands-on care.

Good communication between staff and family members can certainly influence the quality of the relationship between the family member and the person with dementia. When people with dementia enter a care home, the relationships they have with their families can be placed under strain; making relatives feel at ease within the home can help them to maintain the relationship which is so important to both resident and relative. When the quality of communication is less good, the strain on relatives can be increased:

> I'd feel embarrassed if he was untidy or dirty when we got there. We all went to see him on his birthday – it was like a big family outing – and he wasn't very spruce considering it was his birthday. None of them had made an effort or had a cake or… And we were all there as a whole family, taking presents and cards, and we weren't even offered a cup of tea.

Staff can assist the relationship between resident and relative further by responding to relatives' needs for emotional support (see below) and by helping relatives spend enjoyable, engaging time with the person with dementia, perhaps through involvement in supported trips and activities, as discussed in Chapter 4.

The well-being of the person with dementia in a care home depends fundamentally on the relationships care staff develop with the person, as well as on the maintenance of pre-existing relationships with relatives and friends. It is our belief that both these processes require the development of an effective channel of communication between staff and the families or friends of the person with dementia. Indeed, the relationship between staff and families is an important aspect of relationship-centred care, and effective completion of the dementia care triangle (see Chapter 1) is essential to good-quality dementia care. Where the resident has no close family or friends, getting to know them as an individual is still essential, but is much more of a challenge for staff, without access to someone who can fill in the gaps in their life story, their interests, achievements, sadness, preferences and values.

THE ESSENTIALS OF COMMUNICATION

As with any relationship, clear communication between the parties is vital in order to avoid misunderstandings and misperceptions. Ideally, this should begin before the person with dementia moves into the home. Pre-admission contacts and discussions set the scene for what is to follow. They can be helpful in identifying the relative's fears and concerns, and in enabling the relative to learn something of how the home operates and its philosophy.

Communication between the care home and relatives

Communication requires time, so time for relatives must be built into the running of the home. Relatives should be encouraged to ask questions without feeling that they are bothering the staff:

> You have to find the time for the relatives... You couldn't keep this continuous communication – this rapport – if you didn't find the time. (Staff)

Sometimes, staff view relatives as being an additional burden, but there needs to be recognition that they are an integral part of the work of the home. A care home that promotes 'best practice' will have 'working in partnership with families' as part of its regular training programme for care staff; such homes will involve family members in these training sessions, so that there is a real opportunity for staff to reflect on relatives' perspectives.

It is essential that relatives know who they should talk to about any concerns or queries they may have. In some homes this will be the manager or matron. In others, it will be a specific member of staff, a keyworker perhaps, who is responsible for the resident's care plan. This contact person should make efforts to establish good communication with the family and make sure that there are clear arrangements to cover this role when he or she is not on duty. Such arrangements should be clearly stated and made explicit; at a relatives' meeting in one home, the manager asked the dozen or so relatives present to indicate if they knew who their keyworker was – not one relative put up their hand! Keyworkers need time set aside from other responsibilities to have one-to-one meetings with the relative; this might include visiting the relative at home, so that they are on their own territory and can be more at ease.

The home should also keep in regular contact with relatives who live some distance away, or find it difficult to visit for other reasons. This may require the establishing of a range of ways of communicating with relatives, as face-to-face contact is not always possible or convenient. Telephone contact or even e-mail can be a lifeline to people who find it difficult to visit.

As well as time, listening carefully and respectfully is an essential component of good communication. Recognising a relative's needs for emotional support may require a readiness to listen to the unspoken messages, the tone of voice, the sad or worried expression, as well as to what is actually being said. Checking out with the other person that you have understood their meaning, and that they have heard and understood what you are saying, reduces the risk of misunderstandings through lack of clarity or through one or other party making assumptions or jumping to conclusions as to what the person is trying to say. Mutual respect is vital, and can be demonstrated through efforts to spend time with the person and take seriously what they have to say. Trust is a fragile and elusive quality:

it takes time to build up, but can be so easily broken – by a promise not being kept, a confidence being shared without permission – and, once broken, it is difficult to re-build.

Relatives in most homes will have a number of staff with whom they need to communicate, and they should be introduced to new members of staff, not left to work out for themselves who people are and what their role is. Photographs of staff with their names and positions displayed prominently and kept up to date can be a help. Relatives also need to be told about staff changes; when staff go on holiday or leave the home having established a good relationship with the relative, they need to make a point of saying good-bye to residents and their relatives.

Communication within the staff team

Within the staff team there also needs to be effective communication so that information actually reaches the people who need it, whether that is a relative or a particular member of staff. Systems need to be in place to ensure that information is passed on, as appropriate. Hand-over meetings at the change of a shift are very important for informing staff about anything that has happened during the earlier shift. Team meetings are also important forums for managers and staff to share information. The same essential qualities, of dedicated time, efforts to listen carefully, clarity, respect and trust apply to effective communication within the staff team. Without it, the best efforts of some staff members in building relationships with families will be diluted and negated by colleagues lacking necessary information or skills.

SHARING INFORMATION

Sharing information is not simply a matter of having a noticeboard or newsletter for relatives. It is a two-way process, and here we will consider the process from both perspectives, based on the findings of our European research with care home staff and family members. This research indicated that staff and families of people with dementia in care homes each possess knowledge that could be of benefit to one another. Exchanging such information and knowledge is a vital component of any successful partnership, and is particularly important around the time when the person with dementia first enters the home.

What information do staff need?

Many relatives have been the main carer prior to admission. Their experiences of providing up to 24-hour care, often over a period of several years, means that these relatives have a great deal of expertise in caring for the person with dementia. For instance, they may know of interventions or strategies that have been useful in helping to calm the person down, distract them, or persuade them to do something. By asking relatives about their experiences as carers and using this expert-knowledge within a philosophy of partnership, staff will be in a better position to develop a flexible plan of care that is tailored to the individual needs of the person with dementia:

> That's all we knew, that he was married and had a son; that's all we had been told. We didn't even know what his job was. If background information is collected, we never see it. (Staff)

Each person with dementia is unique, shaped by a lifetime of experiences, relationships, choices and preferences. The more information staff have regarding a resident, the more personalised his or her care plan can be. However, people with dementia often enter long-term care at a point when their ability to communicate is impaired, making it difficult for staff to get to know the person and his or her needs. Families are usually a good source of information about their relative with dementia, and they can help greatly by sharing knowledge of the person's life story with the staff. It is essential, however, that people with dementia are encouraged to contribute as much as they are able to this biographical profile, so that their own perspective is not lost entirely:

> Just before my wife went in…the matron came to our house and she had about one and a half hours with her, holding her hand, finding out about her. And I thought that was quite a nice

> gesture really, so she knew who she was, and who was coming in a couple of days later. (Relative)

The process of gathering information about the person with dementia should begin around the time of admission, ideally before the person moves into the home and otherwise during the person's initial assessment. If possible, the person with dementia could be visited at home by the manager or matron of the home prior to the admission. As well as starting the process of information exchange and 'getting to know you', the home visit helps staff to understand the caring context from which the person with dementia is coming. Where prospective residents have a care manager, the home liaises with the care manager about arranging visits prior to the admission. The home should also actively seek information from health and social care services that the new resident has already been involved with.

However, the process of getting to know the resident does not stop at this point, and more details are likely to emerge as trust between relatives and staff develops. As well as enabling staff to personalise the care they give, such knowledge can help them to understand the behaviours and comments of residents. This then helps to enhance the communication between members of staff and the resident.

Information gathering also helps staff get to know the resident's family and to understand the nature of the relationships between the person with dementia and his or her relatives. In particular, staff should explore the understanding of dementia the family already possesses, the context in which prior care has been provided and the impact dementia has had on the family. Armed with this knowledge, staff will be in a better position to support these important relationships:

> Birthdays and anniversaries, they made sure my mum had a card to give my dad...things that were significant for them, they would make sure that she'd made something to celebrate that. (Relative)

It is essential that the home has an effective system for recording residents' biographical information, which can be accessed by the appropriate personnel. All necessary information about a person's needs – such as dietary requirements and personal night-time routines – should be passed to the relevant care and catering staff.

The purpose of gathering information about the resident's life must be kept clearly in mind: it is not to build up a dossier of private or intimate information that the person would not want to be shared; it is to help with communication and to inform and personalise the resident's care plan. As mentioned in the previous chapter, producing a life story book with the person with dementia and his or her family provides a good way of highlighting aspects the resident and family are comfortable to share, and an excellent means for new staff members to get to know the resident, by sitting down together and going through the book with them. The life story book contains pictures and text of important events, roles and people in the person's life. As well as providing staff with valuable information about the person with dementia, the life story book is used for reminiscence purposes and provides an excellent aid to communication. As things may get lost, copies of photographs, newspaper clippings and other material are used rather than the originals. Some relatives will be happy to work on such a book with the minimum of guidance from staff; for others, staff may need to be more pro-active.

Respect for confidentiality is vital if relationships are to flourish, and trust be maintained. Gossip regarding the intimate details of residents' lives is unacceptable inside or outside the care home. In small, rural communities – where residents may have been known to staff for many years before they were admitted to the care home, and staff and residents' lives and families may have points of overlap and interweaving – being clear and explicit about the need to respect confidentiality is especially important.

What information do relatives need?

a) Information about the home

At the time of admission, there will be many sources of anxiety for the relative. This will be heightened by unfamiliarity with the home and its policies – and the resulting uncertainty may increase feelings of loss of control over what is happening. Taking time to show relatives around and introducing them to staff and residents is a first step in helping them adjust to this new environment.

Relatives also need to know what they can do in the home (in terms of visiting, giving assistance to the resident, involvement in decision-making, etc.), as discussed in Chapter 4, and any misconceptions they have should be identified and discussed. It is important, then, that staff spend time giving practical information, answering questions and reassuring relatives. Information about the routines, policies and procedures of the home and other issues affecting residents and their families needs to be written down in a simple pamphlet or brochure and given to prospective residents and families. This information should be reviewed and updated regularly to accommodate any changes. Relatives should be invited to comment on the home's information material, with the home using this feedback to produce more family-friendly material, written in accessible style and language.

Families should be encouraged to visit and seek information about different homes before the decision about the move is made. Relatives of prospective residents could be encouraged to make several informal visits to the home and be put in touch with the families of residents before deciding on which home is most suitable. The greater their knowledge and experience of different homes, the more likely it is that the chosen home will best meet the needs of the person with dementia and his or her relatives. It will also assist the relative to feel some sense of control in the decision-making process. Increasingly, relatives and residents of care homes (both current and prospective) have access to inspection reports produced by the relevant regulating authority; they should be encouraged to read them before making their decision, to obtain an independent view alongside their own subjective impressions.

However, it needs to be recognised that admission often happens in a crisis, when decisions regarding placement are made very quickly, and there is then no opportunity for the family to view a number of homes.

b) Information about dementia

It can be very daunting for families when they see other residents who appear to be at more advanced stages of dementia. Concerns may arise about what further changes they might expect in their own relative, and questions regarding the inevitability of change and the progression of impairments and disabilities are likely to surface. While some relatives have a very good understanding of dementia and how it affects people differently, others may benefit from further information.

Where this need is identified, staff can help by explaining some of the facts about dementia and answering relatives' questions. In order to be in a position to do this, staff themselves need to be well trained in understanding dementia. They may also be able to direct relatives to other sources of information, including literature (books, leaflets, etc.), organisations such as the relevant branch of the Alzheimer's Society, and, perhaps through carer-support programmes, other people who have experience of being a relative of someone with dementia. Gaining knowledge about dementia can help relatives to be prepared for changes they may witness in the future. Staff may also need to help relatives understand and come to terms with changes as they take place.

Families of residents need to be spoken to honestly and realistically, but also with sensitivity. Their need for information will be particularly pressing during the terminal stages of dementia. This sharing of information works best in the context of an established relationship between the staff member and the relative. Sometimes staff can also help relatives to prepare for the death of the resident, and end-of-life issues are discussed in more detail in Chapter 6.

c) Information about the resident's activities and condition

Keeping relatives up to date with what is happening in the home is an important aspect of sharing information. Staff should, of course, keep relatives informed of any significant changes in the resident's health or well-being. Relatives will vary in what they consider to be a 'significant' change, and the home needs to respect these differences. Some relatives will appreciate frequent up-dates, others will be content to be contacted only if there is a major change. The frequency of visits and the closeness of contact will influence these aspects. What is important, of course, is that relatives do not find themselves in the situation of 'discovering' the person has had a fall, or an infection, or a change in medication when they visit, without being pre-warned by the staff concerned.

Relatives may also like to hear about activities in which the resident has been involved since their last contact, and any achievements or pleasurable experiences they may have had, no matter how small. Keeping relatives informed in this way will help them to still feel a part of their loved one's life and may help to make visits more meaningful, giving them topics to talk about. Keeping relatives informed about forthcoming activities, such as trips out, coffee mornings, relatives meetings, etc., is also essential in keeping channels of communication open.

d) Information about family involvement

Care homes should also aim to produce information about the role and value of family involvement within the care home, and how this is appreciated by the care home staff. Contact numbers for the home, personalised information about the 'key staff' involved with their relative's care, timing of relatives' support groups and relatives' management/representation groups, are all important matters to include in such information brochures. It is vital that relatives continue to have a meaningful voice within the organisation of a care home, and open channels of communication (as promoted in this chapter) are the vehicle to drive forward this involvement. Additionally, information available to families should include the contact details of national organisations, such as the Alzheimer's Society (www.alzheimers.org.uk) and the Relatives and Residents Association (www.relres.org.uk), where confidential telephone helpline support can be accessed, and further information found should this be necessary.

SUPPORTIVE COMMUNICATION

Everybody needs support from others from time to time, and this is particularly important for those involved in the care of people with dementia. Relatives will also need support to help maintain their relationship with the person with dementia when he or she moves into a care home and to manage the emotional effect of this new phase of their caregiving career. This section addresses ways in which relatives can be offered the support they need. In Chapter 7, the needs of staff for support in coping with the demands of their work are considered.

Providing emotional support

> I just couldn't cope any more so she went in to the nursing home full time. But the thing that hit me first of all was the guilt – did I do enough and could I have carried on a bit longer? And I didn't get instant relief – I didn't think the weight of the world's been lifted off my shoulders because the guilt cancelled that out. (Relative)

Contrary to popular belief, the problems and worries experienced by families and friends do not instantly disappear when the person with dementia moves into a care home. In fact, staff need to be aware that the problems and worries experienced by families can actually get worse at this point. It's true that there may well be a sense of relief for the relative that the person with dementia will now receive the care that could no longer be provided at home. However, it is also common for relatives to experience a range of negative feelings, including sadness, grief, loneliness, anger, and guilt at having let the person with dementia down. Some people may feel anxious about the quality of care their relative will receive from the care staff. They may also have a sense of helplessness, or loss of control over the person's care. Those who had been the main carer may also be at the point of exhaustion, and have few sources of support left around them.

Staff should watch out for, and be sensitive to, possible feelings of guilt and emotional turmoil that many relatives go through when they place a loved one in care. These feelings can sometimes be expressed as anger or resentment towards the staff. Staff should be calm and clear with relatives to reassure them that they have not failed their loved one. This support can be essential for relatives at this difficult time:

> The problems in the initial months of him going and all the things I was unhappy about, I'm sure they were made worse because I was feeling so guilty. I was thinking I'd let him down. (Relative)

On the other hand, some relatives don't experience these negative feelings when the person with dementia moves into a home. For example, the relationship between the resident and relative may not have been good prior to the move. Staff should therefore not automatically assume that all relatives will feel guilty.

Relatives build up relationships with staff over time. Older spouses who might see themselves as private people may not be comfortable sharing family matters with 'outsiders'. Staff need to be aware that relatives will vary in their willingness to discuss personal feelings with them and that the emotional support required will vary from person to person. Continuity of staffing and an effective keyworker system make it more likely that a supportive relationship can be established.

Admission affects each relative differently, and staff should take the time to ask relatives how they feel about it. Spouses often feel the loss of their partner acutely, especially if they are now living alone for the first time since they were married. They need to know that they are welcome to spend as much time as they want to with their partner, particularly in the first weeks. Intense feelings of loneliness are not unusual at this time.

Adult children, especially daughters, may feel that they have let their parent down, and conflicts can develop between siblings who disagree about the decision to seek long-term care. Staff may need to mediate between relatives to help each of them accept this change in their parent's life. Relatives who have been really worn down by caring may want to distance themselves from the situation for a while. They should be helped to feel that this is acceptable so that they can resume involvement when they feel ready.

Even after the resident settles in, visiting can be upsetting for relatives. It is distressing for them to see deterioration in their loved one's health and abilities, and it is especially hard when the person with dementia no longer recognises them. The resident's behaviour may also be difficult for relatives to cope with during visits. Observing the progress of dementia and disability, and feeling powerless to prevent it, can be a distressing experience for many relatives. Staff who provide a 'shoulder to cry on' in private can be a comfort to distressed relatives. In a good home, staff will regularly provide opportunities for relatives to talk with them at the end of a visit, asking if everything is alright and offering a cup of tea and an opportunity to talk if they seem upset. Staff can also help by putting the person in touch with sources of support and counselling where this is needed.

It is also important, of course, that staff do not thoughtlessly add to the relative's emotional burden. It can naturally be very upsetting for relatives if they witness staff being disrespectful towards residents, ignoring them, using 'baby talk', or shouting at them, apparently assuming they are deaf. This can exacerbate the relative's own feelings of guilt.

Care is also required in informing the relative about incidents in which the person with dementia has behaved in an inappropriate way. For example, if the person has been aggressive to a member of staff or another resident, it is not unusual for a relative to experience feelings of guilt, almost on behalf of the person with dementia. The relative may also have fears that if the person with dementia 'misbe-haves' the home may reject the person, and another care home will need to be found. This fear may be based on the reality that some homes do, indeed, consider certain types of challenging behaviour beyond their competence and capability to manage.

One constructive approach a home can take in such circumstances is to mention the incident to the relative in the context of seeking their advice as to whether such an incident had occurred previously, and on ways the home could learn from the relative about responding to and preventing such incidents. Recognising that there may be a range of reasons for such incidents – including the approach used by staff, and the physical health problems or the effects of dementia in the person with dementia – can help the relative not to take personal responsibility for them. Engaging in clear, open dialogue allows fears and concerns to be discussed openly, and provides the opportunity for the relative to be offered appropriate support.

For many people, their psychological state and well-being fluctuates with the course of the disease in their relative, often on a daily basis. When the person with dementia has a good day, so does the relative, and vice versa. If relatives appear abrasive it could be because their loved one is ill or in pain that day, or some new problem has become apparent. It is important that staff understand the complex relationship between the well-being of residents and that of their relatives:

> The owner of the home my mum was in was super. If he ever saw you looking slightly upset, straight away he was always there, arm round your shoulder, and 'Come and have a cup of tea with me and a chat', that sort of thing – very, very good like that. And, of course, you get friendly with some of the regular staff. And particularly in the last few months of Mum's life, they were brilliant because it was very distressing… There was always somebody coming into the room when you visited to make sure you were okay, and sit with you and have a chat. I felt that they were very supportive. (Relative)

People who experience particular difficulties in their lives often find it helpful talking to others in a similar situation. The relatives of other residents can therefore be another good source of support for families. Contact with other relatives can be useful for sharing experiences, venting feelings, and sharing tips on how to solve problems, as well as helping relatives to feel less of an 'outsider' when they visit the home. Forming friendships in this way can sometimes be very helpful for those who are perhaps feeling socially isolated after years of caregiving at home. Staff can help by introducing visitors to one another when they meet or by organising meetings between relatives. Some homes offer a relatives' support group, enabling families to meet, discuss matters of mutual concern and socialise. This can also be a good forum for introducing education about dementia for families. Alternatively, or in addition, staff may introduce families to a relatives group or association for families of people in care homes, external to the home organisation. In some centres, support programmes for relatives' post-admission distress have been offered, recognising the significance of this issue.

One component of any good relationship is mutual respect and appreciation. In the context of the relationship between the care home and the relative this can influence the degree of satisfaction that relatives derive from their involvement in the home. Relatives need to know that their visits, interest and involvement are appreciated by staff because they may receive little positive feedback from the person with dementia. They also need to know that staff value their opinions; if the relative feels devalued, this will add further to the emotional impact of their situation:

> I would say something about how he used to like something at home, and they would contradict me. It was as if the five years of my looking after him didn't really count... I knew his little funny ways, and I knew that if he was doing a particular thing – because he didn't speak – I knew why he was doing it and what for. I would try and get that across, but it was as if 'Oh, we're the professionals, we know what we're doing'. (Relative)

DEALING WITH CONCERNS, COMPLAINTS AND CONFLICTS

> All sorts of little things were niggling me, and when I went to tell the matron, she changed it round as if *I* was at fault, so we got a bit cross with each other at times. But it's calmed down now – I will accept anything that she tells me, and she will accept anything that I want to do. (Relative)

All effective communication involves careful listening. A good home will therefore welcome suggestions and deals positively with relatives' concerns and complaints by listening carefully and sensitively to them. Relatives themselves also need to have the courage to speak to staff about any concerns they have, so that any issues can be dealt with early on before they become major problems. If staff respond defensively, relatives may then be reluctant to complain for fear that there may be negative consequences for the resident. An inability to be open and discuss concerns in a constructive way will be damaging for staff–relative relationships. In the case of a major problem, there should, of course, be a clear complaints procedure.

In a similar way, the home needs to be open to the concerns of staff who are worried about poor quality of care. Staff often find it difficult to complain, as they may fear losing their job. Again, there must be a positive approach by the management, recognising that care falling below accepted standards is not in the best interests of the home in the long run. The concerns of staff and relatives need to be viewed as opportunities to improve the service to residents. We are considering here a three-way, triangular relationship between staff, relatives and residents. At times, there may be disagreements and apparent conflicts of interest. Staff may feel relatives are not acting in the best interests of the person with dementia. Relatives may feel their loved one's or their own needs are being overlooked.

Even within families there can be some conflict or disagreement. Relatives may disagree about the decision to move the person with dementia into a home. They may also have different opinions about care practices within the home. Staff often need to actively support communication and facilitate negotiation within the family, both before and after the move. A family conference may need to be held when a conflict arises within the family or between relatives and staff, and specialist advocacy services are now available that can assist in such situations. Although there are often no easy solutions to these problems, without clear communication they are likely to escalate and become more difficult to resolve.

Some homes establish a relatives meeting in which concerns can be raised with staff and management, providing a supportive atmosphere within which relatives feel able to contribute. This also allows relatives to be involved in the process of developing or changing care policies. Relatives meet sometimes with, sometimes without, staff present. Such meetings should be distinguished from relatives' support meetings, which have the different, but equally important, purpose of providing support for relatives in managing the impact of having a relative with dementia in a care home.

Homes that are provided by the voluntary sector are sometimes able to arrange for relatives to be represented on the management board of the home, thus having a real say in the operation of the home. It's also a simple matter for every home to have a suggestion box for staff and relatives! The important issue is the commitment of the home management to taking relatives' concerns seriously, and preventing, as far as possible, serious matters of concern and of complaint arising.

CONCLUSIONS

Good communication is clearly vital to establishing and maintaining a strong relationship between staff and relatives, which is central to relationship-centred care. Like all relationships, this needs to be worked at, and involves staff listening to, and taking seriously, the perspective of family members. Exchange of information, and recognising both the expert knowledge of relatives and their information needs, helps to build the relationship. Supportive communication is also needed to assist relatives in managing the emotional impact of their situation. Open, non-defensive communication is needed to assist relatives in voicing their views and concerns, and staff must be ready to respond positively to differences of opinion amongst family members and to complaints and suggestions. There now follows a checklist (Box 5.1) to be used by care homes to review communication systems already in place.

Box 5.1 Checklist on communication

Use the following checklist to review information sharing practices, communication and support systems in this home. If the answer to any of the questions is 'no', possible solutions need to be considered.

Do relatives think that they receive adequate information about the home before admission?

Are relatives given information about the policies, practices and procedures of the home?

Is the written information produced by the home accurate and kept up to date?

Are relatives routinely asked to provide background information about the person with dementia?

Are the relevant members of staff aware of this information and do they use it in caring for the person with dementia?

Do relatives know who to talk to about the care of the resident?

Is it easy for relatives to approach staff for information during visits?

Do relatives feel confident to express worries or concerns with staff?

Do staff feel comfortable about dealing with relatives' worries and concerns?

Does the home have a forum in which staff and relatives can meet to discuss common concerns?

Are relatives and staff aware of the procedures for making complaints?

Do relatives have opportunities to meet with the families of other residents?

Is it easy for relatives to approach staff for support during visits?

Have staff received any training in counselling relatives?

Do relatives feel valued for their involvement in caring for the person with dementia?

KEY POINTS

- Staff need to know about the person with dementia so that they can deal with each resident as an individual and personalise the care they provide.

- Families are a good source of knowledge about the person with dementia and can supplement any information the resident is able to provide.

- Relatives who looked after the person with dementia before he or she moved into the home have a great deal of expertise as carers; their knowledge and skills are valuable assets and should be utilised by staff.

- Families need clear information about the home and its policies in order to avoid misunderstandings.

- Some relatives will also benefit from receiving information about dementia.

- Staff should strive to keep relatives informed about the person with dementia so that they can still feel a part of the person's life.

- Staff should react sensitively to relatives' distress.

- Relatives may benefit from the support of other families.

- Both staff and relatives need to be shown appreciation for their input into the life of the person with dementia.

- There should be clear and effective channels of communication so that information passes easily from staff to relatives and vice versa.

- Complaints procedures should be understood by relatives and staff.

- Relatives and staff should be encouraged to discuss their concerns with the management. Concerns and criticisms need to be dealt with constructively.

- Staff may need to mediate between relatives where there are disagreements about what is best for the resident.

Chapter 6

Family Involvement and End-of-Life Care Issues

This chapter focuses on the end-stages of dementia, which are often accompanied by a range of difficulties, and sometimes distress – for relatives and staff as well as for the person with dementia. Effective communication between relatives and staff remains the central issue, and requires even more attention at this difficult time. The provision of timely, appropriate and relevant information is discussed and we outline ways of involving families in decision-making, in accordance with the wishes of the person with dementia, taking into account any information from a living will, etc. A family-centred approach, driving these other aspects, is described, emphasising inclusion and involvement.

INTRODUCTION

Death is an inevitable part of human existence. For a person with dementia living in a care home, the end of life can be accompanied by many different experiences. These may include: immobility, pain, swallowing difficulties, shortness of breath, dehydration, constipation, urinary incontinence, the fighting of an infection and a struggle to meaningfully interpret, articulate and interact with the outside world. For some, it is a world shrunken to the size of a bed and the view from a pillow.

For the family, a number of emotions and responses may be evoked, ranging from relief and comfort at seeing the end of a loved one's 'suffering', to feelings of bereavement over the loss of a loved parent, partner or spouse; anger over 'the dementia' and its deleterious effect upon human life; guilt at not being able to do more to help; and, possibly, fear over the witnessed death and a hope that 'this is not part of my future'.

For care staff too, end-of-life care for a person with dementia will bring mixed emotions and professional duties. Some feelings may mirror those experienced by the family, particularly sadness over saying a final 'goodbye' to a person who has been present in their lives, and in the life of the care home. Paradoxically, there will also be a need to remain emotionally 'strong' for the family and to be a pillar of support through this difficult time and transition. Moreover, care home staff will also need to perform palliative care responsibilities to the best of their ability during the last days of the life of the person with dementia by tending to their intimate care needs when the person's ability to indicate, for example, levels of pain and pain relief is significantly compromised. It is not the easiest of times, but many care staff also report satisfaction in the performance of these tasks and in the ability to uphold the dignity of the person with dementia during the last days, hours and minutes of their life. There is much to learn and reflect upon in order to facilitate improved care practice.

The end of life of a resident with dementia will also have an emotional, physical and psychological impact upon other care home residents, a 'coming to terms' with loss and a need to deal with emotions. For instance, for other residents this could be in the ending of close friendships, or a need to manage feelings when confronted with a newly created 'space' within the care home environment, such as a previously favoured and occupied chair in the sitting room that now stands vacant: a stark reminder of the passage of time and that nothing stand stills forever. Contemplating our mortality bring us all face to face with a truth that we do usually our level best to avoid.

There are many issues at the end of life, but, in reflecting the focus of this book, this chapter will look primarily at the role of the family at the end of life of a loved one with dementia, and describe some approaches to partnerships that may help in fostering, brokering and supporting this transition. However, to set this discussion in context, we will commence by briefly outlining some basic considerations in end-stage dementia.

WHAT IS END-STAGE DEMENTIA?

At the beginning of this century a study was published by Kay and his colleagues (Kay, Forster and Newens 2000) that showed that around 25 per cent of people with dementia will end their days in a nursing home compared with 56 per cent who will die in hospital. If we consider that, at present, there are over 800,000 people living with a dementia in the UK, then a quarter of this total, 200,000, will die within a dedicated care home setting – and their families will be confronted with decisions around care procedures and practices. That is a lot of people who will be touched by end-of-life issues if we understand the notion of a 'family' to be flexible and consist of more than two people.

It is well known that the severity of the dementia is a major 'risk factor' to entering the end-stage of the condition and in the subsequent need for palliative care interventions. Dementia is typically thought of as progressing through a number of stages: from a state of 'normal' health through to minimal–mild–moderate–severe stages of dementia. In an influential report, the Audit Commission (1999) defined severe dementia as:

> Where the person is totally disorientated, unable to communicate in normal speech, may fail to recognise close relatives, and is incontinent and completely dependent on others for personal care. As the dementia progresses, the person can become immobile and totally physically dependent. (p.9)

Of course, people with milder degrees of dementia do develop, or already have, other illnesses and conditions that can lead to death. But, in talking with care home staff, and through our own exposure to the care home environment, it is clear that even in cases of severe dementia it is difficult to accurately predict the start of the 'end-stage'. Some suggest that this phase may be characterised by the person with dementia's profound weakness, the fact that they are essentially bed-bound, drowsy for long periods, have increasingly less interest in food and fluids, difficulty in swallowing medication and experience a severely limited attention span and disorientation. It is at this time, the day(s) immediately before death, that traditional models of palliative care practice have their place within the care home and where families themselves, should they so choose, will be involved in care delivery.

However, predicting the end of a loved one's life is fraught with difficulty, and defining this precise time in a person's life when they are in these last days will, more often than not, be drawn from the previous experience of care home and medical staff who have witnessed and tended to this process many times before. Nonetheless, however well informed, and however accurate the prediction, this information and preparation of the family may not remove the shock, pain and huge upset that is experienced at this turbulent time. The death of a loved and significant person is not one that can be easily rationalised and explained away. It hurts. And it will continue to do so.

However unpalatable (and as the Audit Commission definition of severe dementia suggests), it is a fact that severe dementia brings with it many complicating and debilitating factors for the individual. The loss of mobility and self-care problems it brings mean that the person may eventually become bed-bound and dependent upon others to meet all their 'basic' human and personal care needs. This state of physical dependency can bring with it many complicating factors such as a heightened susceptibility to fevers and infections, e.g. pneumonia, and also the risk of acquiring pressure sores due to prolonged immobility. The measurement and experience of pain by people with dementia who are unable to clearly articulate its location, and their individual tolerance threshold, is currently subject to much debate and study.

Although this is a complex phenomenon, people with dementia still have the right to pain relief and so the duty is on the care staff, with assistance from the family, to help translate subtle indicators of expressed pain (e.g. hand movements, face twitching, agitated vocalisation, sleep changes) to identifiable levels of suffering. Conducting this procedure to a high and accurate standard with each individual at all times in their journey through the end of life is a difficult task, but the biography of the person with dementia, the expert knowledge of the person held by the family (and care staff should the person have been a resident in the home for some time) and the care staff's sense of 'knowing' should all come into play to help identify need. Neglecting the assessment and treatment of pain in a person with dementia is simply not an option in person-centred practice.

It is also usual for people with dementia to be admitted into a care home when they are in the more moderate/advanced stage of dementia, and, as Margallo-Lana and colleagues (2001) reported, more than 80 per cent of people with dementia living in care homes have behavioural or psychiatric symptoms – with symptoms of agitation, such as aggression and restlessness, occurring in over half this number. Whilst people with dementia cannot be defined solely through their exhibited behaviours, such actions can create care environments that present as challenging for staff, families and residents alike and make it hard to find an overriding sense of peace and tranquillity when a resident with dementia is entering the last few days of their life. There are no simple solutions to creating this environment, but it goes without saying that good staffing levels, access to private space and single bedrooms and well-educated care staff who are known to the person with dementia and their family will ensure that a home is in a prime position to provide a positive caring culture.

FAMILIES AND PEOPLE WITH DEMENTIA: END-OF-LIFE CARE EXPERIENCES

So, what can be done to help minimise this hurt and promote maximum awareness and inclusion of families at the end of life? There is not, of course, one strategy, or approach, that will revolutionise all care practices. However, a combination of approaches, coupled with a strong value-base in the care home that promotes partnerships and positive choice for families, could be a useful starting point.

Specifically, actions with families that address effective communication, information and decision-making and family-centred care may be helpful, and each of these is now addressed in turn.

Effective communication

Effective communication between care home staff, families and the person with dementia is the cornerstone of successful care practice. Communication is heightened when all parties involved in the process have a common purpose, a shared understanding of the language that is being used, and can each apply the meaning of their communication to their individual set of circumstances. When a resident is in the terminal phase of dementia, and challenged by cognitive capacity and deficits in speech and articulation, then the requirement for effective communication between all those involved is intensified, with alternative approaches necessary to include diverse viewpoints.

Interestingly, when families are pressed to recount what they see as important in (professional) care provision at the end of life for a person with dementia, they do not place their own needs at the top of the list. Far more important to families is the caring attitude that is expressed towards the person who is dying and for care staff to be seen to be acting in their 'best interests' and with an informed and 'friendly' demeanour. The communication and 'caring' process by care home staff towards the person with dementia who is dying is seen by families as the primary indicator of quality of care. Specifically, the 'caring' process was exemplified by providing comfort, relieving pain and keeping the person clean and dry whilst, at all times, maintaining a caring attitude. It is informed action towards the person with dementia who is dying, as well as demonstrating compassionate and caring thoughts, that matters most to families.

With ever-changing policy directives and raised societal and consumer expectations about maintaining high-quality care, care home staff can find themselves operating increasingly under a 'blame culture'. This can even lead to some care homes calling an ambulance to take the person to hospital when the end is near: almost as if to show that everything that could be done to prevent the death was done. In fact, this can simply result in a bad death, where the person is separated from the familiar place and people of the care home, in a disruptive series of moves and unfamiliar places. Where there is good, supportive, open communication, preparations can be made, and often families can reach a point of acceptance that death will come, and affirm the importance of a good death.

In a care home setting, it is usually the 'hands-on' care provider, such as the nurse or other care staff, who informs the family that death is imminent when the resident has entered the terminal phase of their dementia. Of course, the person who brings the 'bad news' can be held responsible for that news. As mentioned earlier in the chapter, there may well be an intensive grief reaction expressed by families during the final days of a loved one's life, and also in the days following the death, and it is vital that care staff have the necessary communication, and counselling, skills necessary to facilitate the families' expression of emotions. For some families, the emotions may manifest themselves in upset and anger at 'the dementia' for robbing them of a life with a loved person, both now and in the past – a situation that has been termed 'dual dying' by Jones and Martinson (1992).

Indeed, studies and clinical observations have repeatedly demonstrated a correlation between the experiences of relatives prior to the death of the person with dementia and their reactions after the person has died. At such times people in distress can redirect their anger away from the person with dementia who is dying and direct it towards care staff. Whilst these emotional outbursts can, at one level, be understandable, they can nevertheless be hurtful to care staff who feel that they have done their best to provide care in difficult and distressing circumstances. If such a situation is encountered, it is crucial for care home staff to understand the meaning behind the outburst and to keep it in proportion to the emotional hurt that is being experienced by families. It is also important that care home staff adopt effective and facilitative communication skills, such as listening, giving time and demonstrating a non-judgemental attitude, to help families in their journey through the transition of loss, bereavement and adjustment.

All situations and emotional reactions will be different; for example, some families may experience a sense of guilt over feeling 'relief' that the person with dementia has died and that they are now unburdened from any caring responsibilities, including, it has to be said, financial responsibilities for care costs. Even within families, different reactions may occur – with the surviving spouse feeling guilt over the loss whilst the children, for instance, express relief over the death and a sense of release. What remains constant for care home staff is the forming and forging of care partnerships that are built from a foundation of mutual trust and understanding. As described, the cornerstone of this foundation is effective and meaningful communication, and this communication may well continue long after the person with dementia has died as (some) families wish to keep in touch with the care home and other residents. The bonds that are forged at this time are often remembered for a lifetime and the opportunities that care home staff can create for continuity of support are vital for some people as they adapt to a life without the person with dementia. The 'hole' that can be left in families' lives by the death of a person with dementia should not be under-estimated, and one way of coping with this loss is through the provision of good-quality information. We therefore now go on to consider this issue.

Information and decision-making

At the point of diagnosis of dementia, relatives and people with dementia often come to understand that the eventual destination of the diagnosis is one of palliative and end-stage care. It is probably, subconsciously, a reason why people with dementia who have been diagnosed early in their condition tend to focus on the 'here and now' and let the future 'take care of itself'. However, an opposing view is that the preparation for end-of-life care and choices must start as early as possible, and preferably when the person with the dementia is willing and able to play an active part in the planning and decision-making process.

Living wills are one way of respecting and making real the choices and decisions of people with dementia who have now entered the end-stage of their condition. The legal and ethical/moral framework from which end-of-life decision-making stems is the product of shared, accessible information and care home staff must not be afraid to ask for and distribute such requests. In England and Wales, the provisions of the Mental Capacity Act come into force in 2007, and provide a clear framework for any person who has capacity to appoint a person who will act on their behalf in relation to decision-making about care, if and when the capacity to make such decisions is lost. Advanced decisions to refuse treatment will also enable the person with dementia to specify in advance of losing their decision-making ability how they wish to be treated in particular circumstances.

The availability and accessibility of information also needs to be placed within an overall model of the experience of living with dementia. Early attempts at developing trajectory models of the caring experience for family carers adopted a temporal and adaptive perspective – largely viewing family care as beginning at a pre-diagnostic stage and continuing through to the admission of the person with dementia into a residential-care facility, or to the time of their death. For example, in a classic study, Lindgren (1993) labelled this trajectory as a 'caregiver career' and identified three distinct but overlapping stages:

- an Encounter Stage (the diagnosis and losses of previous life patterns)

- an Enduring Stage (managing extensive care routines and social isolation)

- finally, an Exit Stage (the relinquishment of caring through the death of the spouse, or their admission into care).

Whilst this temporal model has an overwhelmingly negative construction of the caring experience (and one that has been countered by more positive descriptions of its interpersonal dynamics and relationships), there is, nevertheless, an acknowledgement that family care and adjustment moves over time and does not end once 'hands-on' caring ceases. As part of an information-giving strategy, having information available that is built from an understanding of care as experienced by family carers can help to personalise the approach and make it more meaningful to all those involved in the process.

Information is particularly important in the assistance of family carer's decision-making through the 'stages' of a caregiving career. In the 'Exit Stage', it is known that if relatives can accept the diagnosis of the terminal phase and are assisted to then reframe illness-related challenges in more manageable ways – and have positive reinforcement to take on and complete such problem-solving – then the 'stress' associated with living through and witnessing the end of a loved one's life will be reduced.

Acknowledgement of this process is important because it opens the door to exploring the carer's physical, psychological, emotional and social adjustment to end-of-life issues and how these experiences are continually shaped and reconstructed over the course of a caring career. As an illustration, Sweeting and Gilhooly (1990) pioneered the application of the constructs of 'anticipatory grief' and 'social death' to the process of caring and dementia. They noted that, whilst the person was still alive, some carers grieved for the loss of the person they once knew.

Sometimes, from the carer's perspective, the person was effectively 'dead' as the person that had been known, and was now a 'shell' of their former self. They suggested that when relatives are eventually able to discuss the death of their dependent, either real or imagined, they felt 'unburdened' at the ability to share and confide their fears. This 'open disclosure' of loss and emotional dissonance is a subject that is not limited to the family care of people with dementia and has been reported in caring situations where there is prolonged exposure to terminal illness. However, what is important here is that families are provided with information that normalises their emotions and helps to provide levels of security and comfort from the knowledge that they are not alone in working through this situation.

To make the most of each situation, therefore, information should be:

- tailored to fit the needs of families at the time and stage in which they find themselves

- written in a way that is understandable

- available for distribution in a language of choice

- relevant and helpful in clarifying the family role in care and in promoting choice, autonomy and decision-making.

However, providing information is only one part of the story. It is also vital that such information can be absorbed by families, is designed to help the situation faced by families and clearly articulates the partnership model that is key to successful working practice.

Family-centred care

One way of ensuring continuing involvement of families at the end of life is for the care home to be family-centred in its philosophy, from the point of the residents' admission to the end of their life, and beyond. Family-centred care principles at the end of life for a person with dementia have been described previously by Bonjean and Bonjean (1997). These authors suggest that a care home should operate on the premise of inclusivity and that a philosophy of family empowerment, shared decision-making, tolerance, partnership (that includes the person with dementia) and collaborative practice should underscore the relationship. In a family-centred philosophy at the end of life, it is suggested that families be:

- introduced to all members of staff and invited to a 'terminal stage care conference' so that duties and responsibilities are made clear. This would help to clear up any confusion over roles and provide a platform for mutual understanding and togetherness

- encouraged to call the doctor should they be concerned about any observation in their relative, or about pain control

- provided with information about the care home and procedures

- spoken to in a way that avoids euphemisms about the death experience of their loved one

- involved in writing the care plan so that relatives can indicate the level of support and direct care (if any) they wish to provide

- supported as a whole, not as a part. Here, it is suggested that each member of the family is asked directly about the difficulties they anticipate with the impending death and what staff could do to help.

This would appear to be sensible advice, and an inclusive plan at such a sensitive time in the care process may help to provide a context for the care delivery in the final stages of life.

A family-centred philosophy also makes real the previously outlined principles in this chapter and builds upon the need for clear and effective communication skills from staff. It is also important to highlight the fundamental part played by family members, care home staff, other residents and people with dementia in sustaining relationships at this pivotal time. Relationship formation, and the trust between all parties, is the natural foundation for partnership working and a family-centred approach. Moreover, from previous studies on relationships and family carers' decision-making (Walker and Dewar 2001), markers of family involvement can be seen to operate on four levels:

- first, information is shared

- second, families feel included in decision-making

- third, families know that there is someone to contact when needed

- fourth, the service is responsive to family needs.

Following such a 'marker' system may help to clarify quality of care at the end of life, an area we will briefly return to in the conclusion to this chapter. The two-way exchange of information is as relevant at this time as at any other point in the relationship between relatives and staff. The relative's knowledge of the views and beliefs of the person with dementia regarding death and dying will be invaluable, as will their detailed knowledge of the cultural and spiritual background and practices and rituals that will have significance and meaning for the person with dementia.

Naturally, it is vital that following the death of the person with dementia the family are not just left to their own devices and simply allowed to return home. Within a family-centred approach, it is suggested that the care home and the staff offer ongoing support and comfort to the family. This could be provided in the form of:

- specific and ongoing carer support groups

- offering families a role within the care home – for example, in a volunteer role

- encouraging families to join external support agencies, such as the Alzheimer's Society, so that their experience and expertise in care is not lost and continues to be invested for the good of all families affected by dementia

- the care home simply offering to 'be there' should families wish to have a social visit at any time in the future.

There is no 'right way' to do things at this time in a person's life, but the opportunity for families to have a sense of continuity and familiarity is an important part of the acceptance and adjustment process. Ensuring the care home is represented at the funeral can also be an important indication of support for the family, and a mark of the respect held for the person with dementia.

Lack of knowledge and/or training and the absence of a person-centred value-base to support practice is one of the largest hurdles to implementing quality care in the terminal phase of dementia. Alarmingly, few care home staff receive specialist training in terminal care and most care home training is done 'on the job' and by practical demonstration – that is, by one member of staff to another. If staff are not fully prepared for their role in providing care for people with dementia who are dying, then they may be unable to provide necessary support for the person with dementia, relatives and other residents. Perhaps one of the main challenges arising from this area is to raise the profile of the palliative care needs of people with dementia and the concomitant needs of families.

Families, too, need training and support as some of the procedures at the end of life require skill and knowledge that go beyond most people's 'basic' caring skills. It is not a competition as to who can give the 'best' care, rather it is about respecting the wishes of the person with dementia, enhancing the skills of families to provide direct care and support (should they indicate that they desire this), and providing the operational philosophy for all members of the care home and family to work together to pursue a good death. That, in itself, is a measure of success and respect for the final transition in a person's life.

CONCLUSIONS

At present, there is limited knowledge about the subjective experience of dying with dementia, about user and carer participation in palliative care research and about how people with dementia themselves construct the bereavement process should a close family member die. Currently, the literature on 'end-of-life' issues in family and dementia care can be divided into two broad areas.

The first is focused on end-of-life decision-making by family carers for people with dementia living in a care home. As we have seen in this chapter, families should be encouraged to take as active a part as they need to at this time in life; the onus is on care home staff and systems to provide the value-base for this to happen.

The second area, which has only been touched on in this chapter, is about working with families to define and measure outcomes in end-stage dementia, particularly in the measurement of quality of care. This is, perhaps, more of a complex organisational issue, but we are helped in this process by the work of Teno, Landrum and Lynn (1997) in further examining this issue. These authors proposed 13 domains to describe quality of care in end-stage dementia, and these covered: physical and emotional symptoms; survival time; global quality of life; physical function; advance care planning; medical treatments and location of care; provider continuity and skill; family experience; bereavement; cognition; social contact and participation; spirituality; and patient and family satisfaction. Whilst lengthy, this list has the benefit of measuring the impact and transition through the end of life as a partnership, emphasising the value and importance of relationships and advanced decision-making by people with dementia within the overall lived experience. Conducted through a family-centred approach, these domains provide a valuable starting point for the expression of need and care at the end of life.

Finally, there are several areas where further work in end-of-life care is necessary. Many families experience feelings of shock and devastation in response to the death of a person with dementia, and this shock is associated with a lack of expectancy over the timing of the death. It seems important, therefore, that preparation of families through appropriate information and intervention strategies is employed at salient times over the caring career so that the terminal phase is demystified and therefore feared a little less. Also, there is little known about cultural influences on end-of-life care and whether the location of the death experience (i.e. home vs. residential vs. hospital) has any impact on carers' subsequent coping and adaptation patterns. There is also more to be learned from the expert role played by families in caring at home for a person with dementia. End-of-life care in dementia, and the work done by families at this time in a loved one's life, needs to step out of the shadows of the caring experience into centre stage in the sunlight. It is no longer tenable to continue to shield our eyes from the reality of death and its place in our lives and those we love and care about – and exploration of this area needs to be done through a partnership approach.

KEY POINTS

- The end of life, even in severe dementia, is often difficult to predict accurately.

- Staff and families should work together to identify and alleviate pain experienced by the person with dementia.

- Homes should do all they can to respect the wishes of families and operate an inclusive family-centred philosophy.

- The desires of the family (and the person with dementia) need to be discussed and documented early on.

- Information provided for relatives needs to be tailored to the needs of each family.

- Relatives may need additional emotional support at this phase.

- Relatives should be offered accommodation to stay in the home during the final stages if they wish.

- It is important to both staff and residents to mark the death.

- Care staff need support and supervision.

- Responsibilities of homes towards relatives after the death of the resident include:

  - informing the relatives sensitively

  - allowing relatives to revisit the resident's room

  - giving relatives time to clear the resident's room

  - handing over the possessions in a sensitive way

  - offering ongoing support (or signposting to other sources of support).

Chapter 7

Intervention Programmes and Conclusions

This chapter begins by reviewing a number of specific programmes that have been developed internationally to support and involve families in care homes. We return to the 'Senses Framework', described in Chapter 1 as a model for relationship-centred care, in order to consider the varied objectives of these programmes. The important issue of how to provide support for staff in the challenging tasks that they face is discussed. Some recommendations are made for handling the transition and admission to the care home, which may be useful to care home staff seeking to improve practice and collaboration with colleagues working in the community. Finally, we discuss some challenges in relation to the three key areas of relatives' involvement: advocacy; ensuring personalised care; and monitoring of care.

INTRODUCTION

Throughout this book we have attempted to highlight and promote the value of involving families in the lives and daily living routine of relatives living with dementia within a care home setting. We have outlined findings from research studies internationally and from two specific research studies that provide clear indications of the key issues, and we have drawn out practical guidance and recommendations for care home management and staff. We have argued that the integration of family involvement into the operation and management of a care home should be seen as 'the norm' and not as a 'special case'. As we have seen, such a focus is not without its challenges, but relatives of people with dementia who live in a care home are as much a part of its everyday life as those who live and work within it.

In our opinion, what is needed is a philosophy of care that fully integrates families and offers real choices for participation and involvement. Moreover, this integrated philosophy should be offered within a family-centred approach that respects biographies, caring experiences, expertise and existing personal relationships and social networks in the community. Entry into a care home does not have to be the end of the story for the person with dementia and their family, in terms of their relationships and shared background and experiences. Rather, it can be the start of new opportunities and life experiences, a new phase for existing relationships and the possibility of new relationships and sources of support.

In this concluding chapter we have two main aims:

- first, to outline a number of specific intervention/collaborative programmes for families involved in the care of their relative living in a care home, which have been developed and evaluated internationally

- second, to draw together the main themes of the book in the context of relationship-centred care, and specifically to highlight the needs of staff working in care homes for support if they are to be able to play their part in involving and supporting families.

FAMILY INVOLVEMENT: INTERVENTION PROGRAMMES

Groups for relatives

Several types of structured groups for relatives have been developed. Amongst the earliest was the Family Support Group Model, described by Sancier (1984), which comprised four two-hour sessions of in-depth problem-solving for relatives who had placed a relative in a nursing home. Each session centred on a different theme: feelings about placement and their role in the lives of their institutionalised relatives; making visits mutually satisfying; effective advocacy for their relative's care; questions and issues raised by group members. Sancier (1984) argued that the model 'helps families regain a measure of control and decision-making power in the life of their institutionalised relative' (p.64) and that relatives were able to learn new roles. This, in turn, enabled families to become more competent at working with nursing home staff and fostering a partnership in the care of residents.

In the UK, Perkins and Poynton (1990) evaluated the effectiveness of time-limited group counselling for relatives of younger people with dementia residing in hospital. Compared with a control group, relatives who received ten weekly, 75-minute counselling sessions showed significant improvement at the end of the intervention and at three-month follow-up in the following domains:

- morale and well-being

- knowledge about the nature and course of younger-onset dementia

- the number and range of physical and, especially, psycho-social activities performed with the person with dementia.

There was no apparent effect on the proportion of time relatives spent communicating (verbally and non-verbally) with the person with dementia or on the duration or frequency of relatives' visits.

The finding regarding knowledge of dementia is particularly interesting in light of the fact that almost all participants (controls and counselling group) had previously received similar information in written form. This suggests that counselling is a more effective way of getting this type of information across to relatives. The authors proposed that 'relatives needed the supportive environment of the group to be able to fully assimilate and accept the real nature and course of the dementing process' (p.294). The increased engagement of relatives in activities, following counselling, resulted in them eliciting more responses from the person with dementia; this had the effect of reducing relatives' sense of helplessness and the distress they experienced during visits. All group participants reported that it had been very helpful.

The 'Taking Care of Myself' programme was developed by Ducharme *et al.* (2005a, 2005b) in collaboration with a number of female relatives of people with dementia in nursing homes. It is a psycho-educational group intervention comprising ten 90-minute weekly sessions for groups of six to eight relatives. Participants take part in discussions and role-playing and complete written exercises. The core value of the 'Taking Care of Myself' programme (Ducharme *et al.* 2005a) is to empower family members; the relative learns that the perception and meanings of stress can be challenged and managed through a cognitive 'reframing' of stressful events and interaction, considering them in other, less-damaging, ways, so that, ultimately, family members are able to 'take control' of their emotions and the situation. The programme covers six themes:

1. feeling at ease when visiting my relative

2. expressing my point of view to health-care staff

3. avoiding emotional torment

4. dealing with small daily losses and being prepared for the ultimate loss of my relative

5. identifying and calling upon my support network and community services

6. reorganising my life after my relative's institutionalisation and taking care of myself.

The programme has been evaluated in a randomised controlled trial involving 137 daughters of care home residents with dementia (Ducharme *et al.* 2005a, 2005b). Whilst psychological distress was not reduced, daughters did report reduced role overload at the end of the programme, and greater competence and assertion in dealing with health-care staff and in reframing stressful situations. Daughters attending a 'Taking Care of Myself' programme or group sessions run by the Alzheimer's Society reported greater perceived availability of both informal and formal social support, compared with daughters who received no additional intervention. Three months later (Ducharme *et al.* 2005b), it was found that most of these positive changes had been maintained, although there was no longer a difference in role overload.

The Family Visit Education Programme (FVEP), described by McCallion (2005), aims to help relatives find visiting the person with dementia more satisfying and less embarrassing by teaching them skills to use in their interactions with the person with dementia. Four 90-minute group sessions provide the educational input, covering verbal and non-verbal communication, use of memory aids and responding to problem behaviours. Three one-hour family conferences are interspersed with these group sessions. During these sessions, the facilitator observes interactions between the relative and the person with dementia and then provides feedback on positive aspects and areas that could be changed; the relative is then observed attempting to implement a strategy previously taught in a group session, and further feedback is provided. The programme was evaluated in a randomised controlled trial (McCallion, Toseland and Freeman 1999) involving 66 relatives from five nursing homes. The people with dementia whose relatives attended the FVEP showed reductions in problem behaviours and reduced irritability and depression. Relatives' communication with the person with dementia was also judged to be improved. There was, however, no effect on the way in which nurses responded to the residents' behaviour problems.

Whilst an important step forward, these group interventions for relatives tend to focus only on the family and have not directly addressed the need for changes in staff perceptions and behaviours, and unhelpful organisational policies and procedures, highlighted in Chapter 1. They have relied on, for example, relatives being more assertive in order to influence the key relationship between relatives and staff. However, there are now some programmes that seek to work with both relatives and staff.

Groups for relatives and staff

The 'Partners in Caregiving' programme developed in the USA by Pillemer *et al.* (1998) consists of two parallel workshops, one for staff and one for relatives of residents, of seven hours' duration, which cover communication and listening techniques and conflict-resolution skills. The programme then ends with a joint meeting between relatives, staff and administrators, through which the two former groups have the opportunity to influence practices or policy in the care home. This final session is also intended as an empowering exercise and to strengthen relationships between staff and relatives. A full description of the approach is provided by Robison and Pillemer (2005).

A preliminary evaluation of the Partners in Caregiving programme (Pillemer *et al.* 1998) suggested that the programme was perceived positively by both relatives and staff, with most of them reporting improvements in communication with the 'other' group since the training. In particular, recipients noted that they were more able to understand the other group's perspective, and they reported a decrease in conflict with the other group. Changes in nursing home policies and procedures also resulted from the programme. More recently, Pillemer *et al.* (2003) reported the findings of a randomised controlled study of Partners in Caregiving that included over 900 relatives, 600 staff and 20 nursing homes in the USA. Again, the results of this research revealed the positive impact of the programme and that families and relatives with dementia reported less conflict (and potential areas of misunderstanding) with staff as a consequence of participating.

In Sweden, Lundh, Paullson and Hellström (2003) describe forming 'study circles' in seven care homes for people with dementia. Each circle comprised eight participants, with relatives and staff in equal numbers, working together on the 'Partners in Care' training materials, developed during the European project described in Chapter 3 of this book. (*Partners in Care: A Training Package for Involving Families in Care Homes* by Bob Woods, John Keady, Helen Ross and Clare Wenger is available from Jessica Kingsley Publishers.) These include video and text-based resources, involving training exercises, with four themes, each designed to be covered in a 90-minute session. These themes are:

- sharing information

- sharing the care

- developing supportive relationships

- making it work.

Each group made its own decision regarding who would facilitate the circle. Although in most cases a member of staff was nominated by the group, one circle was facilitated by a family member. These facilitators attended a briefing day to be introduced to the themes and the training resources.

The circles were evaluated in two focus group and reflection days at the end of the sessions and six months later, when staff and relatives from all seven homes met together. The benefits of the approach included improvements in communication between relatives and staff and a greater sense of partnership and community. There was greater clarity about roles and joint working. At the six-month evaluation session, progress in implementing action plans varied between homes but in some there were clear examples of new ways of encouraging two-way communication and information sharing between staff and relatives. The need for regular follow-up meetings of the circle in each care home (so that ideas and momentum are not lost, and to involve new staff and families) was evident.

Collaborative working

Aveyard and Davies (2006) describe a two-year action group that involved care staff and relatives of people with dementia living in a nursing home in a large city in the north of England. The overall aim of the project was to explore ways of collaborative working between residents, relatives, care staff and researchers in order to create the 'most positive environment' (Aveyard and Davies 2006, p.96) for people with advanced dementia and their families. The home was a 'teaching' nursing home, in that it provided regular training opportunities for nursing students and other professionals. The researchers used a variety of research methods during their work within the nursing home, including questionnaires, away-days, action sets and follow-up procedures.

Through this hands-on, action-orientated research philosophy, advancements were made in the quality of care and organisational procedures. These included:

- an activities programme that was set up with and for relatives and families

- the introduction of a unifying assessment process

- the employment of a part-time occupational therapist

- the instigation of a quarterly relatives information and support group and quarterly newsletter

- the introduction of a trained dog into the nursing home, as many people with dementia respond well to pets

- the development of a skills profile for each member of nursing staff.

This whole-systems approach to care home development is obviously more in-depth and focused than the other studies reported in the section, and more expensive to introduce, although it does have the benefit of demonstrating improvement in the culture of care as a consequence of such intense involvement. It clearly shows the benefits of fully involving families in efforts to improve the quality and culture of care.

THE SENSES FRAMEWORK

Aveyard and Davies (2006) explicitly used the Senses Framework (Nolan *et al.* 2003, 2006) and the principles of relationship-centred care (Nolan *et al.* 2003, 2006) to inform and steer their collaborative working project. This framework makes clear that all parties have essentially the same needs, expressed perhaps in very different ways, which must be addressed if progress is to be made. The effects on family members of the pioneering examples of systematic approaches to involving families described in this chapter can also be considered in relation to the six senses:

- a sense of *security*: e.g. less conflict with staff (Pillemer *et al.* 2003), less role overload (Ducharme *et al.* 2005a)

- a sense of *belonging*: e.g. greater sense of community (Lundh *et al.* 2003); more connection to informal and formal social networks (Ducharme *et al.* 2005a)

- a sense of *continuity*: e.g. being able to be more involved in physical and psycho-social activities with the person with dementia (Aveyard and Davies 2006; Perkins and Poynton 1990)

- a sense of *purpose*: e.g. working on memory aids for the person with dementia (McCallion 2005)

- a sense of *achievement*: e.g. being able to communicate better with the person with dementia (McCallion *et al.*

1999) and being more competent in dealing with
health-care staff (Ducharme *et al.* 2005a)

- a sense of *significance*: e.g. feeling empowered (Sancier
  1984) and being better understood by staff (Pillemer *et
  al.* 1998).

In this book we have emphasised the position of family members in
the dementia care triangle, and made numerous suggestions and
recommendations for how staff could work more collaboratively in
partnership with them. However, the Senses Framework reminds
us that staff also require support in order to achieve more produc-
tive and satisfying relationships for all concerned.

SUPPORT FOR STAFF

Staff also need a sense of achievement and significance. They may
not receive much positive feedback from residents, and so appreciation shown by families helps staff to feel valued for the work they
do. Relatives need to let staff know what they appreciate as well as
expressing their concerns.

Although they are employed to provide care, most staff
members show dedication and commitment to a job that, judging
by the level of pay commonly given, tends not to be valued in
society. Staff often form close relationships with residents, feeling
almost part of the person's 'extended family'. Relatives therefore
need to recognise that the care and concern shown by staff may be
often deep and heartfelt; to many staff, it is not 'just a job'. It is
particularly important when the person with dementia dies to
remember that the staff also will need understanding and support
as they grieve for the person they, too, have lost, as the following
experiences illustrate:

> You get so involved with the residents, they do become part
> of your family, because you're working with them all the
> time. (Staff)

> Some of the staff are so caring. I think they treat them like their own relations. They seem to form a bond between them, which is nice. (Relative)

Retaining good staff is in the best interests of residents, their relatives and the home. This is more likely to happen if staff feel valued and supported. The work is often demanding; the environment sometimes noisy and stressful; they are often helping people with basic physical functions where maintaining dignity is a real challenge. They regularly have to contend with incidents of aggression and repetitive behaviour, as well as complaints from relatives. Supervision and support from colleagues are essential for dealing with the stressful nature of the job. Good work should be rewarded. Ongoing training in dementia care is essential because staff need the skills to be able to work effectively and with sensitivity in this setting:

> It would be nice if the family actually asked how we felt sometimes, because we never get that... We never get any recognition.

All staff should have opportunities to reflect on their work: supervision, in a group or individual, should not be viewed as a luxury item, but as an essential requirement for staff in dementia care homes. Ongoing education and training in dementia care is similarly essential; it is skilled, complex work, and training can also assist in team building, which is required to underpin the supportive relationships that are required within a home. Above all, staff need appreciation for their input into the life of the person with dementia; management of care homes has a major role to play in this, of course, but effective partnerships with families can add greatly to this recognition and sense of significance. In terms of interventions, those which actually achieve the goal of staff and families meeting together and listening to each other's views and concerns seem to be most likely to achieve the mutual support that makes such a difference.

THE TRANSITION PHASE

This book has specifically focused on the situation of family members *after* the admission of the person with dementia to the care home, as this has been a relatively neglected topic. There is, of course, much that could be said regarding the transition from caring for the person at home to the placement in a care home, and particularly the family member's experience of this transition (e.g. Davies and Nolan 2003, 2004; Ryan 2002; Seddon, Jones and Boyle 2001). There is no doubt that experiences during this time can have a profound effect on how the placement is perceived and how the family member reacts and adapts to it. Too often, the relative is placed under pressure to 'find a home', and the level of support, practical and emotional, in this process can be far from ideal. Many admissions occur in a crisis, and care homes are left, it seems, to start almost from scratch in getting to know the person with dementia and his or her family.

A number of recommendations regarding this transition phase, with relevance for care home managers and staff, emerged from the European project described in Chapter 3 and listed below.

Pre-admission, relatives need information about:

- the selection of a home – including:
  - matching the home to the person with dementia (e.g. culture)
  - staff/client ratios
  - pre-admission brochure
  - inspection reports
  - informal checks
  - contact with relatives of existing residents
- the nature of the contract with the home
- the other residents

- roles and function of staff

- what relatives can and can't do

- therapies/practices within the home

- activities that go on in the home.

Post-admission, relatives need:

- a copy of the contract with the home

- handbook

- information about the illness

- to be involved in personalising the room

- to be involved in the initial care plan.

The home needs information about:

- the person with dementia and the family (including home visit pre-admission)

    o key dates and key people

    o the resident's daily life preferences

    o the resident's life story

    o the history of the caring relationship

    o languages

    o cultural and religious preferences

- tensions between resident and relative regarding the location of the home.

The home should encourage and facilitate feedback at an early stage:

- this requires an openness of the home to constructive criticism

- the home should encourage/facilitate assertiveness from relatives – to stand up for their rights and those of the resident.

Homes need to have dual set of practices and procedures so that they can cope with both emergency and planned admissions.

FINALLY

In this section, we conclude by looking at some future challenges. In Chapter 4 we identified three ways in which families could contribute to the life of the person with dementia in a care home: acting as advocate; ensuring that care is personalised; and monitoring the care provided.

Advocacy and involvement in decision-making will take on a new dimension with the implementation of the Mental Capacity Act (2005) in England and Wales. Decisions regarding care of a person who is unable to make the decision for him- or herself are for the first time within a legal framework; the person may have already made clear what interventions they would refuse, or appointed a relative to act on their behalf. The role of the relative as advocate will become even more important, and will have more recognition. It has been known for some time that a family role in care home decision-making has benefits on a number of relational and inter-personal dimensions. For example, in a study by Rowles and High (1996) family involvement in the ongoing care for their relative served as a biographical link between the previous life 'at home' and the newly acquired identity of a 'care home resident'. This biographical link was crucial in ensuring care home staff intervened on a person-to-person basis, rather than from the inherent power imbalance of staff member to resident.

As well as assisting staff to offer care in a more personalised way, Rowles and High (1996) also indicated that families performed highly personalised, 'special' tasks during their time with their loved one at the care home, such as performing comforting, pampering and monitoring duties. This is an important observation as it parallels the finding that families of people with more advanced dementia living in the community gain great satisfaction from performing such intimate tasks, which help to motivate them to continue in the caregiving role (Nolan and Keady 2001). Such emotional needs and attachments do not stop once the person enters a care home setting; only the context in which care can now be given changes.

Having an opportunity to tend upon a spouse or parent is, arguably, a validating expression of human love and, whenever this is seen to be wanted, it should surely be fostered and encouraged. It should certainly not be viewed as a competitive act that 'takes away' from care staff roles; inclusivity is the watchword in generating successful partnerships. Responding to the family's need to be needed was recently seen by Gaugler *et al.* (2004) as an approach that strengthened family involvement in care homes and enriched the lives of residents. Accordingly, any barriers to the involvement of families in care homes should be removed and the language of partnership, involvement and participation put in its place.

The challenge for the future will be the increasing role of care homes in end-of-life care with people with severe and advanced dementia. Maintaining personhood and personalised care in advanced dementia, where communication and response are difficult to discern and interpret, is no easy task. Homes will need to develop skills in preparing families for the end-stage and terminal phase of dementia so that it does not come as a total shock. Such preparation is seen as a measure of good practice (Robinson *et al.* 2005) although it is necessary for staff to feel competent in this area of care delivery and in facing up to the emotions that such a subject can engender.

The monitoring role within the care home was observed by Sandberg, Lundh and Nolan (2001) and constructed as an act of 'keeping', such as through 'keeping an eye' on the situation. Arguably, this process of 'keeping' is heightened at the time of the admission into the care home when expectations of family involvement are raised and the family's feelings of guilt, loss and uncertainty are at their height. As Davies and Nolan (2004) report, family involvement in a care home is enhanced if family members are, from the outset, able to view themselves as working in partnership with care home staff. An inclusive organisational-care philosophy, therefore, becomes the crucial determinant to the perceived success, or otherwise, of family involvement and togetherness within a care home setting (Weman and Fagerberg 2006). Care homes are increasingly under scrutiny, with continued debate in the UK regarding how those requiring a care home should be funded, and increasing expectations of quality, not matched by increases in the public funds available. Perhaps the key challenge here is to ensure that relatives are fully included from the outset whenever attempts to work on quality improvement are being planned. More and more homes (and groups of homes) are looking seriously at how they can ensure they provide a service of the quality to which they aspire; families need to be seen as key to this process. Ultimately, this could lead to a future where specific family-involvement programmes are no longer needed in care homes, because the whole philosophy reflects a relationship-centred, family-integrated culture. We still have a long way to go!

Further details of the research projects on which Chapters 2 and 3 of this book are based

CHAPTER 2
'Admission into nursing and residential care: developing a proactive response to carers of older people'

Diane Seddon, Institute of Medical and Social Care Research, University of Wales Bangor

Kate Jones, Institute of Medical and Social Care Research, University of Wales Bangor

Mari Boyle, Princess Royal Trust for Carers

Funded by: National Lottery Charities Board, Health and Social Research Programme

Methods relevant to results presented in Chapter 2

In total, 78 family members whose relative had recently been admitted into a residential or nursing home were interviewed about their experiences for this study. In Chapter 2 we use extracts from family members' personal accounts to describe their post-admission roles and responsibilities and explore the contribution they make to the continued care of the person with dementia. Follow-up interviews with 29 family members ten months later describe how the process unfolds over time and allow the complex and dynamic nature of these experiences to be explored.

The sample was recruited from letters distributed by 37 care homes in North Wales, covering rural and urban areas. The age of family members ranged from 53 to 86 years, with an average age of 60. Most (72%) were women, and 60 per cent were sons or daughters of the person admitted, with 15 per cent being the person's spouse. The person admitted had an average age of 86 years (ranging from 65 to 100) and, whilst not all those admitted had a diagnosis of dementia, two-thirds were reported to have significant memory problems. The 29 family members interviewed for a second time after a period of around ten months were selected to reflect the broad range of characteristics of the total sample and included nine daughters, nine sons, nine wives and two husbands.

CHAPTER 3
'The interface between family caregivers and institutional care for people with Alzheimer's disease and related disorders'

Project Partners:
UNIVERSITY OF WALES BANGOR, UK

Bob Woods, Institute of Medical and Social Care Research

John Keady, School of Nursing and Midwifery

Clare Wenger, Institute of Medical and Social Care Research

Helen Ross, Institute of Medical and Social Care Research

NURSING SCIENCE, FACULTY OF HEALTH SCIENCES, LINKÖPING UNIVERSITY AND UNIVERSITY COLLEGE OF HEALTH SCIENCES, JÖNKÖPING, SWEDEN

Ulla Lundh

Ingrid Hellström

DEMENTIA SERVICES INFORMATION AND DEVELOPMENT CENTRE, ST JAMES HOSPITAL, DUBLIN, IRELAND

Brian Lawlor

Mary Drury

DIRECCIÓN GENERAL DE POLITICA SOCIAL, COMMUNIDAD AUTÓNOMA DE LA REGIÓN DE MURCIA, SPAIN

Alicia Sarabia Sánchez

Eva Rubio Fernández

Funded by the European Commission

Methods relevant to results presented in Chapter 3

A variety of methods was used to gather views and opinions from relatives and from staff involved in care homes; these included semi-structured individual interviews, focus groups, a postal survey and consensus meetings where a range of stakeholders met to consider the issues raised. In total, across the four countries, over 60 staff and professionals participated in this process, together with over 100 relatives. Wherever possible, interviews were tape-recorded and transcribed, and detailed notes taken of focus group meetings. The fieldwork data gathered in each country was analysed to identify emerging themes. With the assistance of professionals and experts in the field and appropriate voluntary organisations, these views were then integrated, at consensus meetings, to arrive at a view of the relationship between staff and relatives, to identify opportunities for constructive collaboration and to highlight the obstacles preventing good working relationships.

Commentary on the context of care homes in the four countries

Whilst there are marked differences in context between the four participating countries, with different proportions of older people and different types of long-term care for people with dementia, there are some key elements in common. These include an awareness of an increase in the numbers of people with dementia requiring care and support, related to the already high proportion of older people in Sweden and the UK now being approached in Spain, with Ireland's older population also continuing to grow, from a lower baseline level. The inherent limitations on family care are also acknowledged; some people with dementia do not have available family, others have carers who have health difficulties of their own, and some present difficulties that are very difficult to manage at home. There is also the recognition that providing good-quality residential care is a difficult task, that there is room for improvement in standards and that staff face a difficult task at times.

Part of the problem is the stigma associated with care homes and their predecessors. For example, institutional care for older people in Sweden was developed from the poorhouses at the beginning of the 20th century; in the UK, residential homes developed after the Second World War from the 'workhouse' and hospital wards were often located in former 'lunatic asylums'. This set the scene for negative attitudes towards institutional care, so that in Spain, for example, institutional care is seen as the last resort, associated with feelings of being unloved by relatives. In the UK and Sweden, there has been some softening of attitudes, as a variety of higher quality institutions has developed. Older people are beginning to place more positive value on not being a burden to their family, and this more often now outweighs the dread and fear of the institution.

However, the emergence of a positive view of the contribution of care homes to the overall spectrum of care is not assisted by examples of homes reported in the media where, in Sweden for example, people have to go to bed in the afternoon or cannot get up until noon because of too few staff, or where they have to eat cold food as there are not enough staff for feeding, or where residents wet themselves without being cleaned, with the home smelling of urine. In the UK, similarly, there have been several notorious scandals involving poor care in residential homes and hospitals for older people with dementia. These have involved units run by the NHS and local authorities as well as those from the private sector. In some instances, physical abuse of residents has been reported. Newspapers and TV investigatory pro-grammes feature such scandals from time to time, although the reports from inquiries appear to have much less impact than those involving child care. One such report in Ireland in 2005 led to changes being announced in the regulation of homes. In Spain, there has also been public concern and investigations regarding the infantile treatment of residents and the use of physical and psychological isolation to control behaviour.

It was clear from the fieldwork that involvement of families in care homes has developed further in the UK and Sweden than in Spain or Ireland, where, in long-term care facilities, the divide between staff and families appears generally larger. In the UK, the establishment of the Relatives Association (re-named the Relatives and Residents Association in 1999) has been instrumental in providing a focal point for relatives of those in care homes to share experiences and to work for closer partnership. The development of innovative dementia care in Sweden and the UK in response to the earlier ageing of the population in these two countries appears to be another important factor. By contrast, in Spain, long-term care facilities for people with dementia are a much more recent development. This is not to say that the UK and Sweden have ideal systems for staff and families to work together. In fact, it is rather that they have more experience and awareness of the tensions that may arise in this relationship.

References

Almberg, B., Grafstrom, M., Krichbaum, K. and Winblad, B. (2000) 'The interplay of institution and family caregiving: relations between patient hassles, nursing home hassles and caregivers' burden.' *International Journal of Geriatric Psychiatry 15*, 931–939.

Aneshensel, C. S., Pearlin, L.I., Mullan, J.T., Zarit, S.H. and Whitlatch, C.J. (1995) *Profiles in Caregiving: The Unexpected Career.* San Diego: Academic Press.

Audit Commission (1999) *Forget Me Not.* London: Audit Commission.

Aveyard, B. and Davies, S. (2006) 'Moving forward together: evaluation of an action group involving staff and relatives within a nursing home for older people with dementia.' *International Journal of Older People Nursing 1*, 2, 95–104.

Bonjean, M.J. and Bonjean, R.D. (1997) 'Working With the Family.' In C.R. Kovcach (ed.) *Late-Stage Dementia Care – A Basic Guide.* London: Taylor and Francis.

Brooker, D. (2004) 'What is person-centred care in dementia?' *Reviews in Clinical Gerontology 13*, 215–222.

Buck, D., Gregson, B.A., Bamford, C.H., McNamee, P., Farrow, G.N., Bond, J. and Wright, K. (1997) 'Psychological distress among informal supporters of frail older people at home and in institutions.' *International Journal of Geriatric Psychiatry 12*, 737–744.

Davies, S. and Nolan, M.R. (2003) '"Making the best of things": relatives' experiences of decisions about care home entry.' *Ageing and Society 23*, 429–450.

Davies, S. and Nolan, M.R. (2004) '"Making the move": relatives' experiences of the transition to a care home.' *Health and Social Care in the Community 12*, 6, 517–526.

Department of Health (2003) *National Minimum Standards for Care Homes for Older People.* (3rd edn). London: Department of Health.

Dobbs, D., Munn, J., Zimmerman, S., Boustani, M., Williams, C.S., Sloane, P.D. and Reed, P.S. (2005) 'Characteristics associated with lower activity involvement in long-term care residents with dementia.' *Gerontologist 45*(Special Issue 1), 81–86.

Ducharme, F., Levesque, L., Lachance, L., Giroux, F., Legault, A. and Preville, M. (2005a) '"Taking care of myself": efficacy of an intervention programme for caregivers of a relative with dementia living in a long-term care setting.' *Dementia 4*, 1, 23–47.

Ducharme, F., Levesque, L. Giroux, F. and Lachance, L. (2005b) 'Follow-up of an intervention programme for caregivers of a relative with dementia living in a long-term care setting: Are there any persistent and delayed effects?' *Aging and Mental Health 9*, 5, 461–469.

Garity, J. (2006) 'Caring for a family member with Alzheimer's disease: coping with caregiver burden post-nursing home placement.' *Journal of Gerontological Nursing 32*, 39–48.

Gaugler, J.E. (2005) 'Family involvement in residential long-term care: a synthesis and critical review.' *Aging and Mental Health 9*, 105–118.

Gaugler, J.E., Anderson, K.A., Zarit, S.H. and Pearlin, L.I. (2004) 'Family involvement in nursing homes: effects on stress and well-being.' *Aging and Mental Health 8*, 1, 65–75.

Jones, P.S. and Martinson, I.M. (1992) 'The experience of bereavement in caregivers of family members with Alzheimer's disease.' *IMAGE: Journal of Nursing Scholarship 24*, 3, 172–176.

Kay, D., Forster, D. and Newens, A. (2000) 'Long-term survival, place of death, death certification in clinically diagnosed pre-senile dementia in Northern England.' *British Journal of Psychiatry 177*, 156–162.

Kitwood, T. (1997) *Dementia Reconsidered: The Person Comes First.* Buckingham: Open University Press.

Lindgren, C.L. (1993) 'The caregiving career.' *IMAGE: Journal of Nursing Scholarship 25*, 3, 214–219.

Lundh, U., Paullson, A. and Hellström, I. (2003) 'Forging Partnerships in Care Homes: The Impact of an Educational Intervention.' In M.R. Nolan, U. Lundh, G. Grant and J. Keady (eds) *Partnerships in Family Care: Understanding the Caregiving Career*. Maidenhead: Open University Press.

Macdonald, A., Carpenter, G.I., Box, O., Roberts, A. and Sahu, S. (2002) 'Dementia and use of psychotropic medication in non-"Elderly Mentally Infirm" nursing homes in South East England.' *Age and Ageing 31*, 58–64.

Margallo-Lana, M., Swann, A., O'Brien, J., Fairbair, A. *et al.* (2001) 'Prevalence and pharmacological management of behavioural and psychological symptoms amongst dementia sufferers living in care environments.' *International Journal of Geriatric Psychiatry 16*, 39–44.

McCallion, P. (2005) 'Supporting Families of Persons with Dementia living in Nursing Homes: the Family Visit Education Program.' In J.E. Gaugler (ed) *Promoting Family Involvement in Long-term Care Settings*. Baltimore: Health Professions Press.

McCallion, P., Toseland, R.W. and Freeman, K. (1999) 'An evaluation of a family visit education program.' *Journal of American Geriatrics Society 47*, 203–214.

Nolan, M. and Keady, J. (2001) 'Working with Carers.' In C. Cantley (ed) *A Handbook of Dementia Care*. Buckinghamshire: Open University Press.

Nolan, M.R., Grant, G., Keady, J. and Lundh, U. (2003) 'New Directions for Partnerships: Relationship-centred Care.' In M.R. Nolan, U. Lundh, G. Grant and J. Keady (eds) *Partnerships in Family Care: Understanding the Caregiving Career*. Maidenhead: Open University Press.

Nolan, M., Brown, J., Davies, S., Nolan, J. and Keady, J. (2006) *The Senses Framework: Improving Care for Older People Through a Relationship-Centred Approach*. Sheffield: University of Sheffield.

Perkins, R.E. and Poynton, C.F. (1990) 'Group counselling for relatives of hospitalised presenile dementia patients: A controlled study.' *British Journal of Clinical Psychology 29*, 287–295.

Pillemer, K., Hegeman, C.R., Albright, B. and Henderson, C. (1998) 'Building bridges between families and nursing home staff: The Partners in Caregiving Program.' *Gerontologist 38*, 499–503.

Pillemer, K., Suitor, J., Henderson, C.R., Meador, R. *et al.* (2003) 'A cooperative communication intervention for nursing home staff and family members of residents.' *Gerontologist 43*(Special Issue II) 96–106.

Port, C.L. (2004) 'Identifying changeable barriers to family involvement in the nursing home for cognitively impaired residents.' *Gerontologist 44*, 770–778.

Port, C. L., Zimmerman, S., Williams, C.S., Dobbs, D., Preisser, J.S. and Williams, S.W. (2005) 'Families filling the gap: comparing family involvement for assisted living and nursing home residents with dementia.' *Gerontologist 45*(Special Issue 1), 87–95.

Ritchie, K. and Ledesert, B. (1992) 'The families of the institutionalized dementing elderly: a preliminary study of stress in a French caregiver population.' *International Journal of Geriatric Psychiatry 7*, 5–14.

Robinson, L., Hughes, J., Daley, S., Keady, J., Ballard, C. and Volicer, L. (2005) 'End-of-life care and dementia.' *Reviews in Clinical Gerontology 15*, 135–148.

Robison, J. and Pillemer, K.A. (2005) 'Partners in Caregiving: Cooperative Communication between Families and Nursing Homes.' In J.E. Gaugler (ed) *Promoting Family Involvement in Long-term Care Settings*. Baltimore: Health Professions Press.

Rowles, G.D. and High, D.M. (1996) 'Individualizing care: family roles in nursing home decision-making.' *Journal of Gerontological Nursing 22*, 3, 20–25.

Rubin, A. and Shuttlesworth, G.E. (1983) 'Engaging families as support resources in nursing home care: Ambiguity in the subdivision of tasks.' *Gerontologist 23*, 632–636.

Ryan, A. (2002) 'Transitions in care: family carers' experiences of nursing home placement.' *Nursing Times Research 7*, 324–334.

Sancier, B. (1984) 'A model for linking families to their institutionalized relatives.' *Social Work 29*, 63–65.

Sandberg, J., Lundh, U. and Nolan, M.R. (2001) 'Placing a spouse in a care home: the importance of keeping.' *Journal of Clinical Nursing 10*, 406–416.

Scottish Executive (2004) *National Care Standards: Care Homes for Older People.* Edinburgh: Scottish Executive.

Seddon, D., Jones, K. and Boyle, M. (2001) 'Admission into nursing and residential care: developing a proactive response to carers of older people.' *Final Report to the National Lotteries Board, Health and Social Research Programme.* Bangor: Institute of Medical and Social Care Research.

Seddon, D., Jones, K. and Boyle, M. (2002) 'Committed to caring: carer experiences following the admission of a relative into nursing or residential care.' *Quality in Ageing 3,* 16–26.

Schwartz, A.N. and Vogel, M.E. (1990) 'Nursing home staff and residents' families role expectations.' *Gerontologist 30,* 49–53.

Sweeting, H.N. and Gilhooly, M.L.M. (1990) 'Anticipatory grief: a review.' *Social Science Medicine 30,* 10, 1073–1080.

Teno, J.M., Landrum, K. and Lynn, J. (1997) 'Defining and measuring outcomes in end-stage dementia.' *Alzheimer Disease and Associated Disorders 11,* 6, 25–29.

Tornatore, J.B. and Grant, L.A. (2002) 'Burden among family caregivers of persons with Alzheimer's disease in nursing homes.' *Gerontologist 42,* 497–506.

Walker, E. and Dewar, B.J. (2001) 'How do we facilitate carers' involvement in decision-making?' *Journal of Advanced Nursing 34,* 3, 329–337.

Welsh Assembly Government (2004) *National Minimum Standards for Care Homes for Older People.* Cardiff: Welsh Assembly Government.

Weman, K. and Fagerberg, I. (2006) 'Registered nurses working together with family members of older people.' *Journal of Clinical Nursing 15,* 281–289.

Whitlatch, C.J., Schur, D., Noelker, L.S., Ejaz, F.K. and Looman, W.J. (2001) 'The stress process of family caregiving in institutional settings.' *Gerontologist 41,* 462–473.

Woods, B. (1999) 'The person in dementia care.' *Generations 23,* 3, 35–39.

Woods, B. and Matthison, G. (1996) *Report on a Postal Survey of Members of the Relative's Association Having Relatives/Friends in Residential Care.* Bangor: DSDC Wales.

Woods, R.T. and Macmillan, M. (1994) 'Home at Last? Impact of Local "Homely" Care on Relatives of People with Dementia.' In D. Challis, B. Davies and K. Traske (eds) *Community Care: New Agendas and Challenges from the UK and Overseas.* Aldershot: Ashgate.

Yamamoto-Mitani, N., Aneshensel, C. and Levy-Storms, L. (2002) 'Patterns of family visiting with institutionalized elders: the case of dementia.' *Journal of Gerontology: Social Sciences 57B,* S234–S246.

Zarit, S.H. and Whitlatch, C.J. (1993) 'The effects of placement in nursing homes on family caregivers: short and long term consequences.' *Irish Journal of Psychology 14,* 25–37.

Zimmerman, S., Sloane, P.D., Williams, C.S., Reed, P.S. *et al.* (2005) 'Dementia care and quality of life in assisted living and nursing homes.' *Gerontologist 45*(Special Issue 1), 133–146.

Subject Index

Author Index